INTRODUCTION

The Federation of State Medical Boards and the National Board of Medical Examiners established the Step 3 examination of the United States Medical Licensing Examination (USMLE) as a single, uniform examination for medical licensure. This test provides a standardized evaluation system to assess the current competence of physicians applying to general, undifferentiated medical practice in the United States of America. The examination consists of four booklets of multiple choice questions. These questions evaluate several aspects of medical knowledge, the understanding of basic and clinical mechanisms of disease, as well as, the cognitive abilities required by physicians in general practice. The most important assessment is directed toward the critical abilities required for diagnostic and management of clinical problems.

ITEMS USED IN THESE BOOKLETS ARE CURRENTLY USED TO PREPARE AND INSTRUCT STUDENTS AND PHYSICIANS AT THE TEXAS TECHNICAL HEALTH SCIENCES CENTER AND THE MEDICAL COLLEGE OF WISCONSIN.

Fourth Edition,
2000 by MAVAL PUBLISHING, INC. Denver, Colorado
Printed in Chile

10 9 8 7 6 5 4 3 2 1

The MAVAL MEDICAL EDUCATION board, expends great efforts to make unambiguous, and medically accurate questions. However, new information may make a previously correct answer to an item incorrect, or may be a source of ambiguity not previously visualized. If inaccuracies and ambiguities occur, consult your references. Because, some items are essential in the learning process, they are being used in one or more of the books and booklets of MAVAL PUBLISHING, INC. In addition, the review of some questions are omitted because the item being covered may not need further review.

USMLE step 3

CLINICAL SCIENCES

BOOKLET C TEST 1

Questions: 94 Time: 105 minutes

Items 1-4

A 59-year-old white male is seen in the clinic for impotence. He has been married for 30 years with two children. He has a history of noninsulin dependent diabetes mellitus, hypertension and depression. He is taking diabeta 20 mg/day, lisinopril 10 mg/day and aminotryptilin 75 mg/day. He complains of a constant inability to initiate and maintain an erection, and a decrease in penile turgidity. His libido is normal. He does not have nocturnal erections and these symptoms have gradually worsened in the past two years.

1. The most likely cause of this clinical picture can be explained by:

a) complications of diabetes mellitus
b) drug effects
c) vascular disease in diabetes mellitus
d) autonomic complications in diabetics
e) all of the above

2. The history is NOT compatible with:

a) psychogenic
b) hypogonadism
c) an autonomic dysfunction
d) a thyroid insufficiency
e) an endocrinology disorder

3. The most appropriate laboratory tests that should be ordered include the following, EXCEPT:

a) serum prolactin
b) serum testosterone levels
c) CAT scan of the chest
d) glycosilated hemoglobin
e) creatinine and BUN in serum

4. Which of the following interventions is NOT indicated in this case?

a) Discontinuation of the offending drug
b) Hormonal replacement if necessary
c) Discuss possibility of a penile prosthesis
d) Castration
e) Reassurance

5. Which of the following tests is useful to evaluate an immune deficiency state?

a) Liver function tests
b) Total lymphocyte count
c) Vitamin B12
d) Calcium and phosphate concentration
e) Chest x-ray

Item 6

A 62-year-old white female is seen in a routine physical examination. She is asymptomatic and in good health, except for constant tiredness. Physical examination is unremarkable, no lymphadenopathy are palpable, and the liver and spleen are normal in size. A complete blood count shows: WBC 345,000/uL, hemoglobin 11.8 mg/dL and platelets 98,000/uL. The blood smear is shown in the figure C.1.

6. The most likely diagnosis is:

a) acute myelogenous leukemia
b) acute lymphocytic leukemia
c) hairy cell leukemia
d) chronic lymphocytic leukemia
e) chronic myelocytic leukemia

Items 7-8

A 39-year-old male complains of enlargement of both breasts with mild tenderness and no discharge. He has a history of testicular trauma, and alcohol abuse. He has taken ibuprofen for years for back pain. The physical examination is remarkable for symmetric enlargement of both breasts with an induration of the right testes.

Prolactin level in serum:	normal
Testosterone in serum:	normal
Cortisol random sample:	normal
CT scan of the brain:	normal

7. The most likely diagnosis is:

a) drug-induced gynecomastia
b) hCG-secreting testicular tumor
c) prostatic carcinoma
d) testosterone insufficiency
e) hyperprolactinoma

Figure C.1

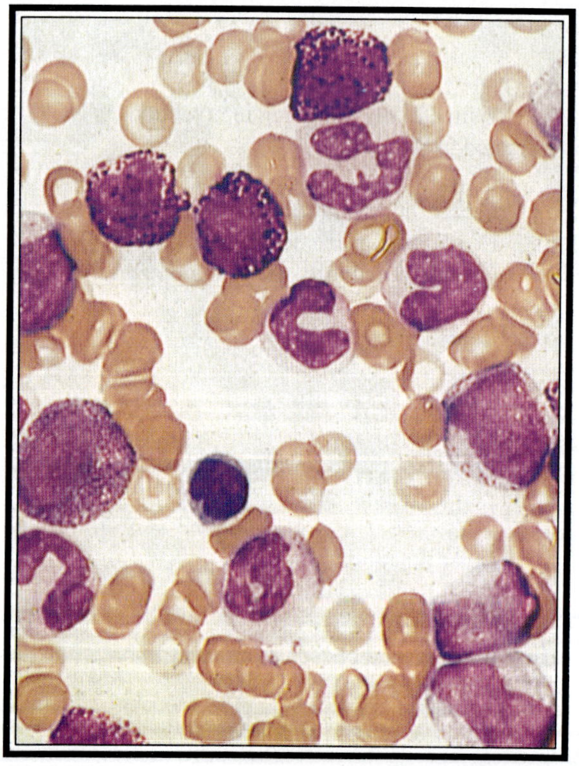

Figure C.2

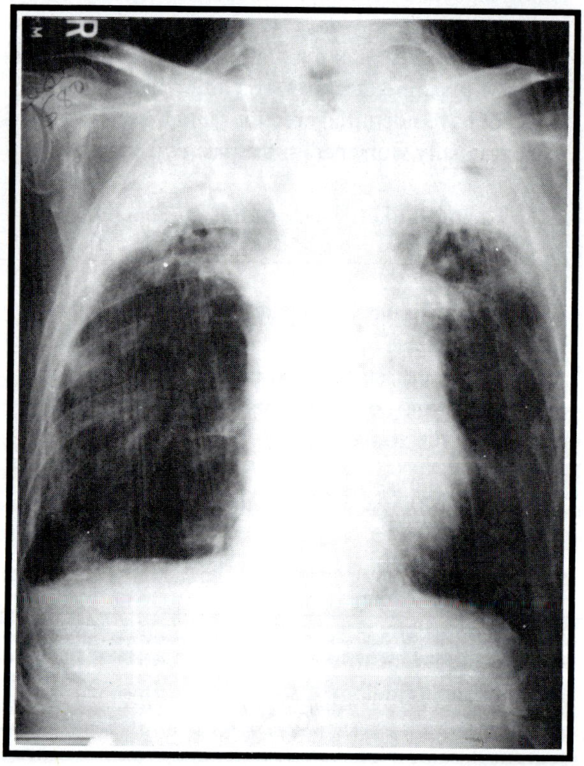

8. Therapeutic interventions in this condition should include the following, EXCEPT:

a) offending drugs should be discontinued
b) antiestrogens
c) monthly testosterone injections
d) treatment of the underlying disease
e) formal breast examinations

Items 9-10

A 42-year-old black male worker in a welding company complains of several weeks of a painful red eyes with photophobia and loss of visual acuity. The examination of the eyes showed a slight ciliary flush, small poorly reactive pupils, and a hazy anterior chamber with flare visible on slit-lamp examination.

9. The most likely diagnosis is:

a) iritis
b) retinal detachment
c) corneal ulcer
d) acute glaucoma
e) UV light conjunctivitis

10. Adequate therapeutic interventions may include the following, EXCEPT:

a) ophthalmologist evaluation
b) topical steroids to reduce inflammation
c) dilatation using hematropine (1-5%)
d) laser therapy
e) evaluation for systemic diseases

Items 11-14

A 32-year-old hispanic male complains of 2 months of non-productive cough. During the last week he had a cough and hemoptysis on two occasions and he is loosing weight quickly (20 pounds in 4 months). He is a non-smoker and he has family history of TB. The physical examination shows evidence of malnutrition, BP 100/50 mm Hg, and a decrease in lung sounds with fine crackles in both apices. The laboratory tests show hyponatremia (129 mEq/L), hyperkalemia (5.2 mEq/L) with lymphopenia (600/uL). Chest x-ray was obtained (see figure C.2)

11. The most likely diagnosis is:

a) sarcoidosis
b) tuberculosis
c) lung carcinoma
d) aspergillosis
e) none of the above

12. The most common underlying conditions and diseases that should be considered in patients with this disease are the following, EXCEPT:

a) chronic bronchitis
b) AIDS
c) silicosis
d) patient treated with immunosuppressive drugs
e) hematologic malignancy

13. The treatment should include:

a) chemotherapy
b) antibiotics
c) prednisone 1 mg/k/day po
d) surgical lobectomy
e) gammaglobulins

14. The abnormalities shown in the serum of this patient is most likely the result of:

a) kidney failure
b) thyroid involvement
c) SIDAH
d) Adrenal insufficiency
e) pituitary involvement

Item 15-16

A 60-year-old white male is scheduled for an elective inguinal hernia repair. He has a history of lung disease treated with beta-adrenergic inhalers and prednisone. His pre-operative laboratory test results are:

pH	7.42	
pO2	61	mm Hg
pCO2	56	mm Hg
Bicarbonate	25	mEq/l
Tidal Volume	300cc	
Minute Volume	6,000	cc
FEV1	1,200	cc
Vital Capacity	3,900	cc
Residual Volume	175%	
DLCO	70 %	

After broncodilator inhalers, vital capacity and FEV1 did not change.

15. Which of the following factors is the BEST predictor of a lung dysfunction in the postoperative period?

a) History of COPD
b) Vital capacity
c) CO2 retention
d) Hypoxemia
e) DLCO

16. Which of the following is most likely the underlying pulmonary disease or functional abnormality?

a) COPD with moderate obstructive airway disease
b) COPD with severe obstructive airway disease
c) Restrictive lung disease
d) Asthma
e) None of the above

Items 17

A 45-year-old white male is seen in the clinic for a physical examination. He denied any symptoms. He is non-smoker and he is taking no medications. The physical examination is normal, except for a skin lesion (see figure C.3)

This lesion is associated with:

a) Polycystic ovarian disease
b) Polycystic kidney disease
c) Neurofibromatosis
d) Polyposis of the colon
e) Chron's disease

Item 18

A 60-year-old white male is seen in the clinic for the lesion on his forehead. He has had this lesion for at least 8 months characterized by a thick adherent scale (see figure C.4). The most likely diagnosis is:

a) Psoriasis.
b) Actinic keratosis
c) Squamous cell carcinoma
d) Giant comedone
e) Keratoacanthoma

19. Which of the following etiologies is LEAST likely to be a cause of habitual abortion?

a) Cervical incompetence
b) Uterine anomalies
c) Uterine retroflexion
d) Infection
e) Genetic errors

Items 20-22

A 49-year-old white male is seen in the emergency room for palpitations, «pounding» chest pain and one episode of syncope. He has been seen prior to this admission for mild arterial hypertension without pharmacological treatment. He is a nonsmoker and he does have a family history for coronary artery disease. His physical examination is remarkable for a harsh systolic murmur in the left sternal border that increases after changing positions (from sitting to standing). An electrocardiogram was obtained (see figure C.5).

20. The clinical and electrocardiographic findings are compatible with:

a) hypertrophic obstructive cardiomyopathy cardiomyopathy
b) hypertensive
c) aortic stenosis
d) aortic insufficiency
e) mitral insufficiency

21. Patient should be treated with:

a) beta adrenergic blocker agents
b) digital
c) diuretics
d) procainamide
e) nitrates

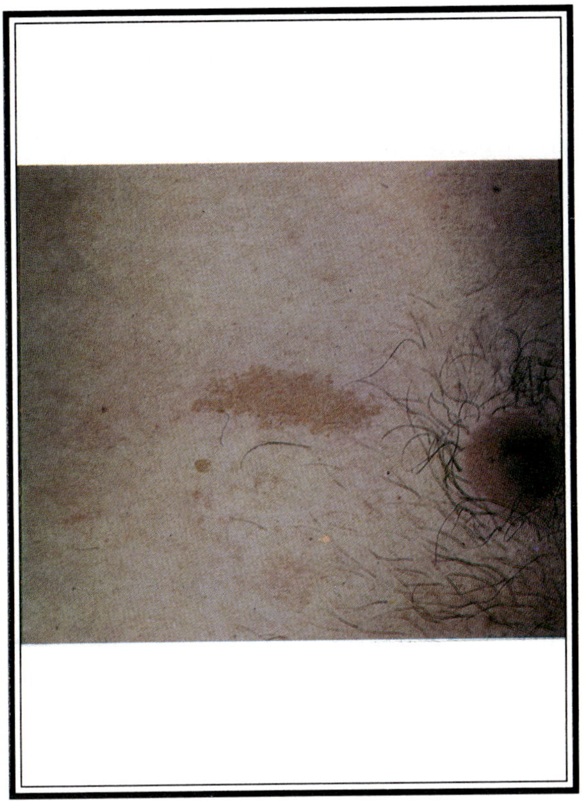

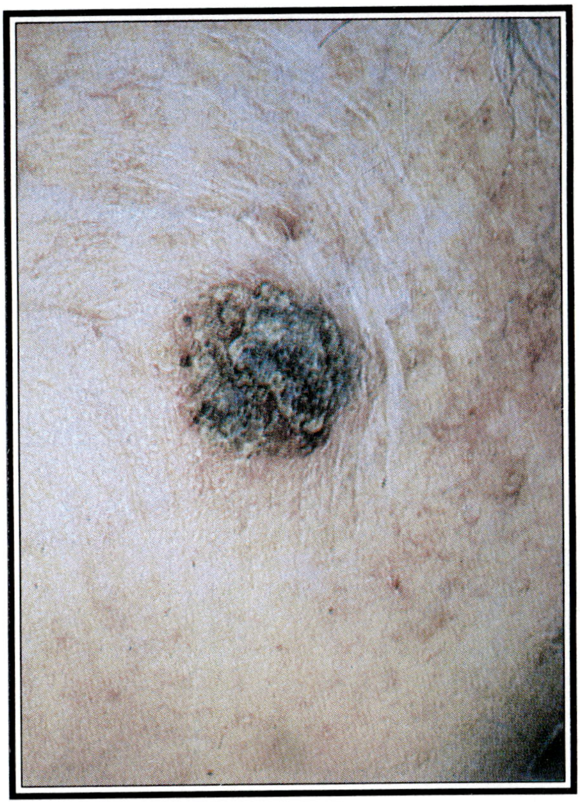

Figures C.3, C4 (top) and C5 (bottom).

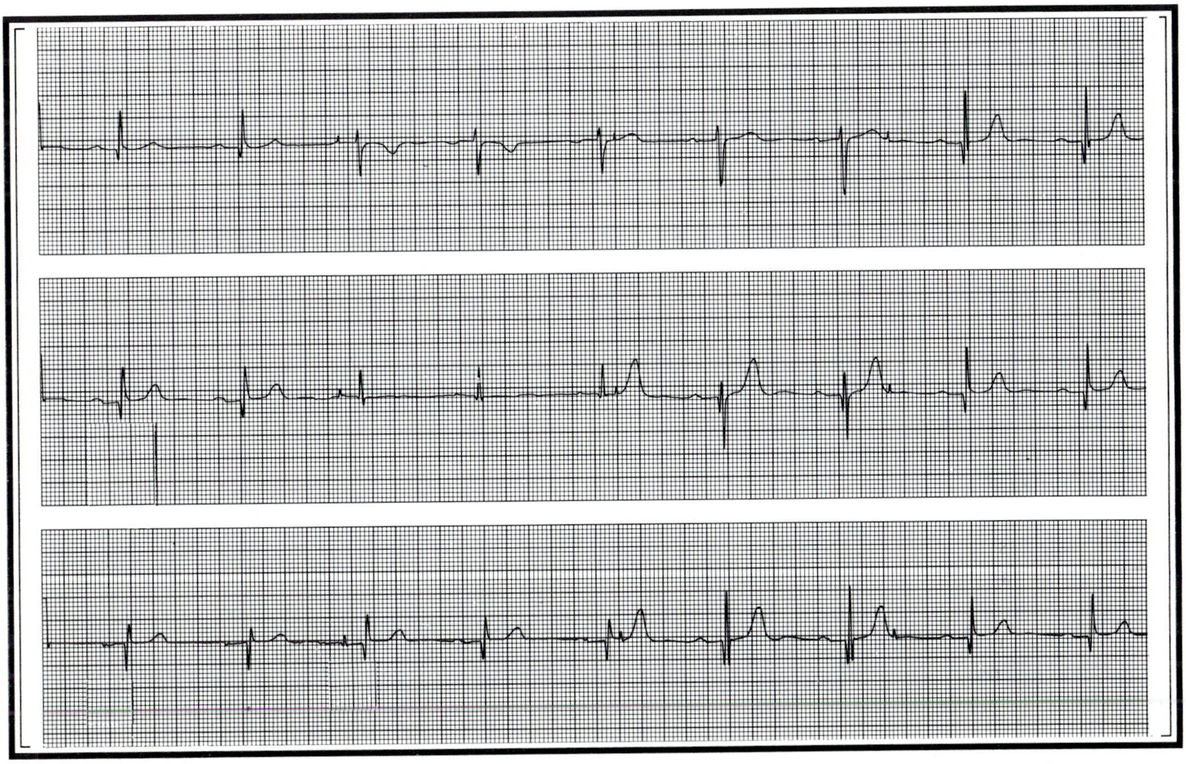

22. Which of the following statements regarding this disease is INCORRECT?

a) Systolic function is usually normal
b) Increased LV stiffness results in elevated diastolic filling pressures
c) Dyspnea on exertion, angina, presyncope and sudden death may occur
d) Symptoms can be improved with positive inotropic drugs and vasodilators
e) Echocardiogram shows systolic anterior motion of mitral valve

23. Auer rods are seen in the smear of patients with:

a) acute myelogenous leukemia
b) chronic myelocytic leukemia
c) chronic lymphocytic leukemia
d) acute lymphoblastic leukemia
e) polycythemia vera

24. All of the following disorders are associated with peripheral blood eosinophilia, EXCEPT:

a) asthma
b) Loffler's syndrome
c) fibroplastic eosinophilia
d) myxedema
e) parasitic infections

25. The early symptom of spinal cord compression (epidural compression) caused by a disseminated carcinoma with bone metastasis is:

a) numbness
b) pain
c) incontinence
d) stiffness
e) none of the above

26. The most appropriate treatment in patients presenting with evidences of spinal cord compression caused by tumor is:

a) dexamethasone i.v.
b) chemotherapy
c) prednisone 60 mg p.o. day
d) laminectomy for decompression followed by chemotherapy
e) none of the above

27. In a patient with recent diagnosis de superior vena cava syndrome, the procedure LEAST useful in the diagnostic work-up is:

a) thoracotomy
b) mediastinoscopy
c) thoracocentesis if pleural effusion is present
d) myelography
e) CT chest

28. The most frequent malignancy that causes hypercalcemia is:

a) prostate
b) breast
c) hepatoma
d) Paget's disease
e) melanoma

Items 29

A 3-year-old child presents with anemia, reticulocytosis, polychromasia and nucleated red cells in the peripheral smear. Neutrophil and platelet counts are normal. The most likely diagnosis in this child is:

a) leukemia
b) anemia in chronic infection
c) hemolytic anemia
d) aplastic anemia
e) erythroleukemia

30. Which of the following is the LEAST likely a neonatal complication seen in diabetic mothers?

a) Respiratory distress syndrome
b) Hypoglycemia
c) Poor feeding
d) Hypercalcemia
e) Hyperbilirubinemia

31. Which of the following is the LEAST common side effect of benzodiazepines?

a) Anterograde amnesia
b) Withdrawal syndrome
c) Respiratory depression
d) Renal failure
e) Paradoxic agitation

Items 32-33

A 4-day-old infant presents copious oral and pharyngeal secretions causing airway obstruction and respiratory distress. The nurse was unable to pass a nasogastric tube into the stomach.

32. The most likely diagnosis of the above clinical presentation is:

a) achalasia
b) esophageal atresia with tracheoesophageal fistula
c) hiatal hernia with gastroesophageal reflux
d) pyloric stenosis
e) none of the above

33. The most appropriate treatment for this infant is:

a) balloon dilatation
b) constant suction and surgical repair
c) surgical reparation of the hernia
d) definitive gastrostomy
e) none of the above

34. Strokes that occur as a complication of myocardial infarct:

a) are usually associated with aspirin treatment
b) are caused by emboli arising from left ventricular thrombi
c) strike in 50% of the patients during the acute myocardial infarct
d) are increased in patients treated with thrombolysis
e) none of the above

35. Which of the following is NOT a feature of the pulmonary hypoplasia in newborns?

a) Severe respiratory distress
b) Small lungs are seen in the chest-x-ray
c) Large thoracic cage is seen in chest-x-ray
d) Pneumothorax, pleural effusion or both
e) Early hypoxemia

Items 36

A 6-year-old child presents with pica, apathy, lethargy, ataxia, vomiting and seizures. He lives in an old house where his father has a small factory of lead-glazed ceramic pots. Laboratory shows hemoglobin 9 mg/dl and hematocrit 28% with an increase in free erythrocyte protoporphyrin. The most likely diagnosis in this patient is:

a) Wilson's disease
b) paraquat intoxication
c) lead poisoning
d) porphyria
e) none of the above

Items 37-40

Identify the following diseases with its clinical presentations.

a) Marfan's syndrome
b) Tay-Sachs disease
c) Phenylketonuria
d) Galactosemia
e) None of the above

37. Inborn error of carbohydrate metabolism. After milk feedings the infants present hepatomegaly, vomiting, amino aciduria, and growth failure.

38. Autosomal recessive disorder seen most frequently among ashkenazi jewish families.

39. Most common amino acid disorder due to a deficiency of a hydroxylase enzyme. Dietary restrictions can avoid mental retardation.

40. A disorder of the connective tissue resulting in long, thin limbs, scoliosis, pectus excavatum, hypermobile joints.

41. Which of the following is LEAST likely to be seen as intracranial complication of an acute sinusitis?

a) Meningitis
b) Malignization
c) Cavernous sinus thrombosis
d) Subdural empyema
e) Brain abscess

42. Genetic disorders that most likely cause mental retardation are the following, EXCEPT:

a) phenylketonuria
b) mucopolysaccharidoses
c) Alport's syndrome
d) fragile X-syndrome
e) galactosemia

43. True statements regarding the antipsychotic drugs are the following, EXCEPT:

a) chlorpromazine has significant hypotensive side effects
b) thioridazine may present minimal extrapyramidal side effects
c) trifluophenazine and fluphenazine have the least sedative and hypotensive side effects
d) trifluophenazine and fluphenazine have the highest extrapyramidal side effect
e) chlorpromazine has minimal sedative side effect

Items 44-45

An 80-year-old patient with sundown syndrome, congestive heart failure and COPD complains of dry mouth, constipation and urinary retention. He is taking several drugs including isordil 30 mg t.i.d., aspirin, capoten 25 mg t.i.d, theophylline 300 mg b.i.d. and chlorpromazine 500 mg q.d. He is seen in the clinic where his blood pressure was 130/90 mm Hg, pulse 75 bpm regular and involuntary movements of the jaw are seen in the physical examination. No other neurological abnormalities are seen.

44, The involuntary movements of the jaw or tardive dyskinesia is most likely the side effect of

a) isordil
b) chlorpromazine
c) aspirin
d) capoten
e) theophylline

45. The indication of antipsychotic drugs in this patient is to treat:

a) the urinary retention
b) the involuntary movements
c) the agitation seen in the elderly
d) the symptoms of the sundown syndrome
e) none of the above

46. What is the most frequent cause of non-streptococcal pharyngitis in young children?

a) Adenovirus
b) Mycoplasma pneumoniae
c) Influenza virus
d) Parainfluenza virus
e) None of the above

47. Which of the following statements regarding streptococcal pharyngitis is INCORRECT?

a) 20-40% of the cases are caused by group A streptococci
b) Penicillin can prevent acute rheumatic fever
c) Children with positive throat cultures should be treated with antibiotics for 10 days
d) It can cause pneumothorax, empyema and purpura with disseminated intravascular coagulation
e) It is most common in children and young adults

48. Which of the following is the most frequent cause of acute diarrhea in infants?

a) Irritable bowel disease
b) Systemic infection
c) Gastroenteritis
d) Antibiotic associated
e) Improper feeding

49. Idiopathic nephrotic syndrome of childhood is a disorder characterized by the following, EXCEPT:

a) proteinuria
b) hypoproteinemia
c) hyperlipidemia
d) hematuria
e) edema

50. Children with vitamin D deficiency may present the following, EXCEPT:

a) normal or low calcium level in serum
b) low serum level of phosphorus
c) low serum level of alkaline phosphatase
d) osteoporosis
e) rickets

51. The major cause of hemolytic anemia in neonates is:

a) maternal-fetal blood group incompatibility
b) hereditary red cell enzymatic defect
c) thalassemia
d) sickle cell anemia
e) none of the above

Items 52-54

A 40-year-old construction worker, fell from the second floor. He was awakened but he is still drowsy. Bartter's sign was positive. He has no previous medical history. A skull-x-ray was taken (see figure C.6).

52. In the roentgenogram it is possible to identify:

a) frontal and basilar skull fractures
b) a bi-orbital fracture
c) an ethmoidal fracture
d) parieto-temporal fractures
e) none of the above

53. To classify this patient in the «high mortality group» your findings should be the following, EXCEPT:

a) depressed level of consciousness clearly not due to alcohol, or drugs
b) focal neurological signs
c) palpable depressed fracture
d) associated metabolic disorder
e) air-fluid level in the sphenoid sinus seen on the brow-up lateral film

54. Appropriate therapeutic interventions may include:

a) admission in a critical care unit
b) CT scan of the head
c) neurosurgical consultation
d) monitor level of consciousness
e) all of the above

55. Listeria monocytogenes:

a) can cause meningitis and sepsis
b) is a gram-negative bacteria
c) must be treated with a specific antitoxin
d) is transmitted by mosquitos
e) should be treated for 7 to 10 days with ampicillin

Figure C.6

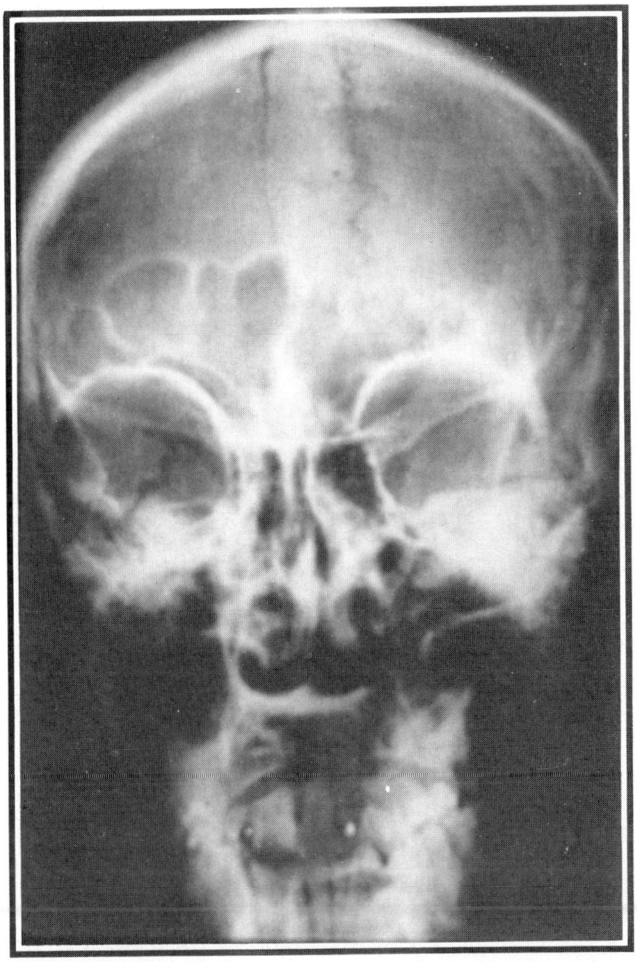

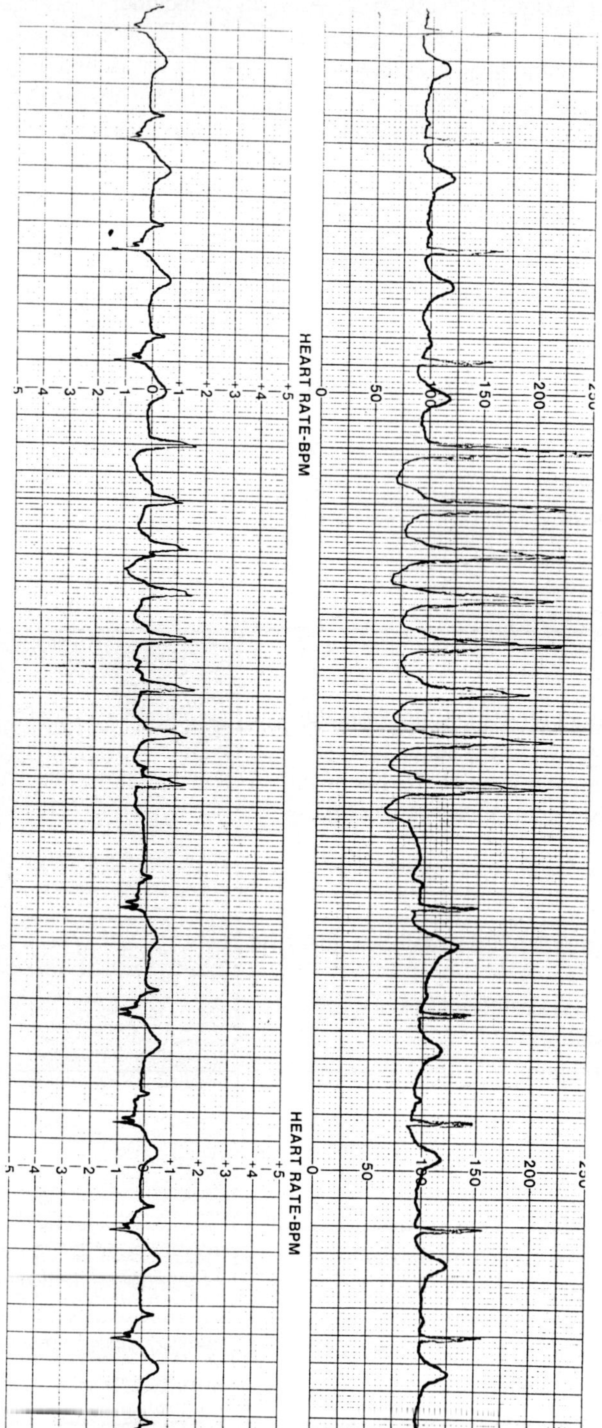
HEART RATE-BPM
0
50
100
150
200
250
-5
-4
-3
-2
-1
0
+1
+2
+3
+4
+5
HEART RATE-BPM
0
50
100
150
200
250
-5
-4
-3
-2
-1
0
+1
+2
+3
+4
+5

Figure C.7

56. A 24-year-old white male is seen for fever (101°F), pain in his right cheek, purulent nasal discharge and postnasal drip. He also complains of several days with morning cough and halitosis. The most likely diagnosis is:

a) dental abscess
b) acute sinusitis
c) acute laryngitis
d) streptococcal pharyngitis
e) none of the above

Items 57-61

Match the features of the cerebrospinal fluid (CSF) with the most likely clinical diagnosis.

a) Bacterial meningitis
b) Viral meningitis
c) Cryptococcal meningitis
d) Tuberculosis meningitis
e) Subarachnoid hemorrhage

57. Comatous patient with abundant red blood cells and white cells count of 1,000 /uL in the CSF.

58. AIDS patient with increased protein (80/mg/dl), WBC 500/uL, predominant lymphocytes and positive serologic test.

59. A 9-year-old boy presents malnutrition, low degree of fever, weakness and lethargy. Lumbar puncture shows CSF pressure 250 mm H2O (elevated); leukocytes 200/uL, 80% PMN; protein 200 mg/dL (elevated); glucose 30 mg/dL (low).

60. A 12-year-old black girl presents generalized weakness, headache, fever and lethargy. Lumbar puncture shows normal CSF pressure; leukocytes 50/uL, 60% mononuclear cells; normal protein and normal glucose concentration. Serological tests are negative.

61. A-4 year-old boy presents fever (103.5°F) and lethargy. Lumbar puncture shows CSF pressure 250 mm H2O (elevated); leukocytes 2,000/uL, 90% PMN; protein 300 mg/dL (elevated); and glucose <20 mg/dL (low).

Item 62-64

A 71-year-old white female is in the critical care unit after having severe chest pain and shortness of breath. She was treated with thrombolysis using streptokinase, aspirin, beta adrenergic blocker and nitroglycerin in continuous infusion. The pain was relieved but she started to feel dizzy with changes in her mental status. The monitor in the unit shows the following rhythm (see figure C.7). Her BP is 120/70 mm Hg, pulse 175 bpm regular, with an S4 heart sound and few bibasal fine crackles in both lungs.

Laboratory analysis:

BLOOD		
Sodium	138	mEq/L
Potassium	4.3	mEq/L
Glucose	170	mg/dL
CPK	430	U/L
CPK-MB	54	U/L
LDH	210	U/L
SGOT	80	U/L
SGPT	56	U/L
WBC	9,600	cells/uL
Hemoglobin	13	mg/dl
Platelets	190,000	platelets/ul

62. The rhythm shown in the monitor is:

a) atrial fibrillation
b) wondering pacemaker
c) ventricular tachycardia
d) torsades de Pointes
e) none of the above

63. The first choice of management is

a) lidocaine i.v.
b) cardioversion
c) amiodarone
d) discontinue the thrombolytic therapy
e) brethylium

64. This arrythmia is most likely caused by:

a) cardiac failure
b) rupture of the myocardium
c) reperfusion in ischemic tissues due to the thrombolysis
d) side effects of the nitroglycerin
e) side effects of beta adrenergic blocking agents

Items 65-69

Match the following seizure disorders with its most common clinical presentation.

a) Grand mal seizures
b) Absence seizures
c) Partial complex seizures
d) Pseudoseizures
e) None of the above

65. It is usually idiopathic with typical sequence of tonic-clonic events and postictal effects.

66. It is often gradual, presenting bizarre actions and behavior with no evidence of biting or incontinence.

67. It is an abrupt onset of seizures with no postictal effects. It should be treated with ethosuximide.

68. It presents a sudden onset of unresponsiveness with staring and postictal effects. Automatisms are seen during the period of unresponsiveness. Treatment usually includes phenytoin and/or tegretol.

69. This seizure disorder usually requires no anticonvulsivant therapy.

70. The most common postoperative complication in diabetic patients is:

a) pneumonia
b) hypoglycemia
c) dehydration
d) renal failure
e) cardiac failure

Items 71-74

A 12-hour-old infant is seen for cyanosis. The Apgar scores were 8 and 9 at 1 and 5 minutes. Apparently, he has never been pink since he was delivered. He weighed 3,300 g at birth. His heart rate is 130 per minute and respirations are 60 per minute. The lungs are clear and no retractions on inspiration are noted. The heart sounds are normal. Pulses are strong and equal and there is no organomegaly. The hands, feet and tongue are dusky and the infant's color darkens when he cries.

Laboratory Analysis:

ABG'S (room air)

pH	7.40	
PO2,	30	mm Hg
PCO2	32	mm Hg

ABG'S (breathing 100% Oxygen)

pH	7.39	
PO2	31	mm Hg
PCO2	33	mm Hg

71. Which of the following tests is NOT indicated in the diagnosis of this infant's disease?

a) Chest x-ray
b) EKG
c) Complete blood count
d) Cardiac catheterization
e) Lumbar punction

72. The most likely disease in this infant is:

a) idiopathic respiratory distress syndrome
b) polycythemia vera
c) cyanotic congenital heart disease
d) systemic hypertension
e) acrocyanosis

The patient heart catheterization was performed and the results are shown in the following table:

	Pressures (mm hg)		Oxygen saturation (%)
Right Ventricle	70/5	Right Atrium	30
Aorta	70/40	Left Atrium	96
Left Ventricle	30/6	Right Ventricle	35
Pulmonary Artery	25/10	Left Ventricle	90
		Aorta	38
		Pulmonary artery	92

73. According to the data obtained from the cardiac catheterization, this child may have:

a) tetralogy of Fallot
b) tricuspid atresia
c) transposition of great vessels
d) normal heart
e) congenital lung disease

74. Which of the following interventions is recommended?

a) Steroids i.v.
b) Mechanical ventilation
c) Aspirin
d) Septostomy
e) Anticoagulation

75. Which of the following recommendations is appropriate in a surgical patient with a history of adrenal insufficiency?

a) To discontinue intravenous fluids the day of the surgery
b) To decrease the maintenance doses of cortisol to one half, the day of surgery
c) To give an intramuscular doses of cortisol (100 mg) just before the operation
d) To administer an intravenous ACTH dose the day before surgery
e) None of the above

76. Oncogenes:

a) are present only in neoplastic or tumoral cells
b) are able to induce malignant transformation of cultured cells
c) contain a viral genome incompatible with the human DNA
d) are only DNA viruses
e) none of the above

Items 77-80

A 9-year-old white boy is seen in the clinic because of a persistent skin lesion on his chin. His mother said that the lesion has been itching with mild soreness (see figure C.8). She also stated that he is her only child and he has been healthy, except for one or two episodes every year of sore throat and otitis. His physical examination is unremarkable except for the skin lesion.

77. Which of the following is the most likely diagnosis?

a) Herpes simplex
b) Cellulitis
c) Erysipela
d) Impetigo
e) Folliculitis

78. The following are significant laboratory findings, EXCEPT:

a) ASO titer elevations are low or absent
b) anti-DNAase B and antihyaluronidase increase significantly
c) total serum complement activity is low during initial stages of acute nephritis
d) sedimentation rate does not correlate with the activity of the disease
e) cultures of the pharynx and any skin lesion may be positive for group A streptococcus

Figure C.8

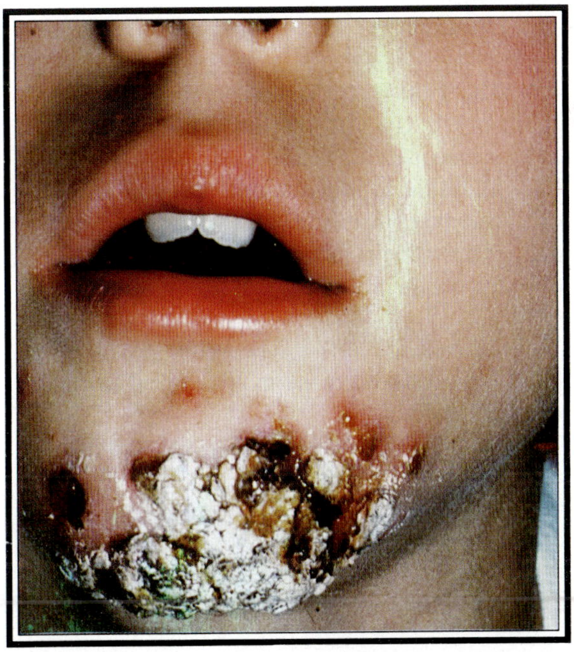

79. Which of the following statements regarding this disease is INCORRECT?

a) These lesions may occur after a minor skin injury
b) Acute neuritis and postherpetic neuralgia are more common in children
c) The disease is self limiting
d) Untreated it may last for weeks or months
e) Rheumatic fever is a common complication

80. Which of the following is NOT a recommended therapeutic intervention?

a) Triple antibiotic ointments
b) Mechanical debridement of crusts
c) Antibacterial soaps
d) Cephalexin p.o.
e) Steroids p.o.

Items 81-84

A 65-year-old white male complains of fatigue, weakness, anorexia, nausea and vomiting with loss of weight. He has had a history of tuberculosis many years ago. His blood pressure is 90/50 mm Hg and the physical examination is remarkable for hyperpigmentation of the skin in areas exposed to sun and knuckles, toes, knees, and elbows. Oral mucosa is also hyperpigmented.

81. The most likely diagnosis in this patient is:

a) paraneoplastic syndrome
b) idiopathic hyperpigmented syndrome
c) chronic primary adrenocortical insufficiency
d) reactivation of tuberculosis
e) hypothyroidism

82. Differential diagnosis in this clinical setting should include:

a) autoimmune disease
b) tuberculosis
c) sarcoidosis
d) Addison's disease
e) All of the above

83. Which of the following findings suggest tuberculosis as a cause of this disease?

a) Positive AFB in sputum
b) Calcification in pulmonary lymph nodes
c) Calcification of suprarenal glands
d) Positive antibodies against hormonal tissues
e) Positive PPD

84. Fludrocortisone should be given to patients with:

a) primary adrenocortical insufficiency
b) secondary adrenocortical insufficiency
c) Tuberculosis pulmonar and ACTH deficiency
d) sarcoidosis and suprarenal insufficiency
e) diabetes insipidus and ACTH deficiency

85. Schmidt's syndrome is associated with:

a) hypothyroidism
b) pituitary insufficiency
c) renal failure
d) hyperprolactinemia
e) iron deficiency anemia

86. The preparation for surgery in patients with hyperthyroidism may include the following, EXCEPT:

a) to infuse an alpha-adrenergic agent the morning of the surgery
b) pre-treatment with propylthiouracil
c) to administer an adequate sedation
d) pre-treatment with potassium iodide
e) pre-treatment with propranolol

87. Reasons for the substantial growth in health care expenditures include the following, EXCEPT:

a) improvements in mother-child health services
b) increasing average age of the American population
c) advances in technology
d) adoption of Medicare and Medicaid to the health system
e) the increase in life expectancy

Items 88-89

Match the features of the following diuretics with its mechanisms of action.

a) Thiazides
b) Acetazolamide
c) Furosemide
d) Spirolactone
e) None of the above

88. It is a weak diuretic inhibitor of carbonic anhydrase which inhibits the exchange of H+ for Na+ in proximal convoluted tubule.

89. It inhibits the Na+/K+/Cl- co-transport in ascending loop of Henle resulting in retention of Na+, Cl- and water in the tubule.

90. The «locked in syndrome» is characterized by the following, EXCEPT:

a) sudden onset of apparent unresponsiveness without warning due to paralysis
b) patients are aware of the surroundings and the conversations
c) in most cases the cause is an infarct or hemorrhage in the temporo-occipital cortex
d) patients may communicate with eye blinks and vertical eye movements
e) patients seem to be comatose

91. Which of the following features of the diarrhea and malabsorption in patients with chronic pancreatitis is INCORRECT?

a) Increased neutral fat (triglyceride) in the stool can be detected microscopically or biochemically
b) The D-xylose test is positive in patients with pancreatic exocrine insufficiency
c) The secretion stimulation test becomes abnormal when more than 75% of pancreatic function is lost
d) Diarrhea is frequently but not invariably associated with pancreatogenous steatorrhea
e) Most patients with steatorrhea respond to replacement of pancreatic enzymes

92. Which of the following statements regarding portal hypertension is INCORRECT?

a) In portal hypertension the average of portal pressure is 20 mm Hg
b) It is caused by increased resistance to portal blood flow
c) Alcoholic cirrhosis causes a presinusoidal obstruction.
c) The most common cause is cirrhosis of the liver
d) Laennec's cirrhosis accounts for 85% of cases of portal hypertension in the U.S
e) In children, extrahepatic portal venous occlusion is the most common cause of portal hypertension

93. Females taking oral contraceptives:

a) develop carcinoma from normal breast tissue
b) increase the incidence of nonmalignant breast disease
c) may not increase the risk of endometrial cancer
d) may increase the risk of developing hepatocellular adenoma
e) none of the above

94. The Child's classification in patients with portal hypertension and liver failure, establish:

a) an additive clinical parameter to determine the severity of diseases caused by chronic ethanol abuse
b) that class A has a bad prognosis
c) those in Child's class C are high-risk patients with correspondingly higher operative mortality
d) an additive clinical and laboratory parameters to determine the probability of renal failure
e) none of the above

USMLE step 3

CLINICAL SCIENCES

BOOKLET C TEST 2

Questions: 95 Time: 105 minutes

1. Sexual activity:

a) is inhibited most of the time in diabetic patients due to functional factors
b) is usually normal in chronic renal failure
c) is inhibited after the intake of large amounts of alcohol
d) usually decreases with the intake of a small amount of alcohol
e) none of the above

Items 2-5

A 34-year-old white male complains of scratching pain on his penis. The physical examination is normal, except for the lesions shown in the figure C.9). He is married and he is currently having occasional intercourse with his pregnant wife who is in her 34th week of pregnancy.

2. These lesions are compatible with:

a) condyloma acuminata
b) syphilis
c) herpes simplex infection
d) granuloma inguinale
e) chlamydia trachomatis infection

3. Which of the following tests is the most useful in the diagnosis of this disease?

a) Thayer-Martin cultures
b) VDRL
c) Direct visualization of the vesicle's content
d) Clinical judgement and occassionaly viral cultures
e) Blood cultures

4. The treatment may include:

a) acyclovir
b) neomycin
c) gancyclovir
d) amantadine
e) bactrim

5. Which of the following statements is INCORRECT?

a) Organisms are usually present in the lesions during the first week of infection
b) Infection in the newborn is associated with more than 5% mortality rate
c) Reinfections are common
d) Acyclovir is a safe drug during pregnancy
e) Immune-suppressed patients are prone to develop extensive local disease and systemic dissemination

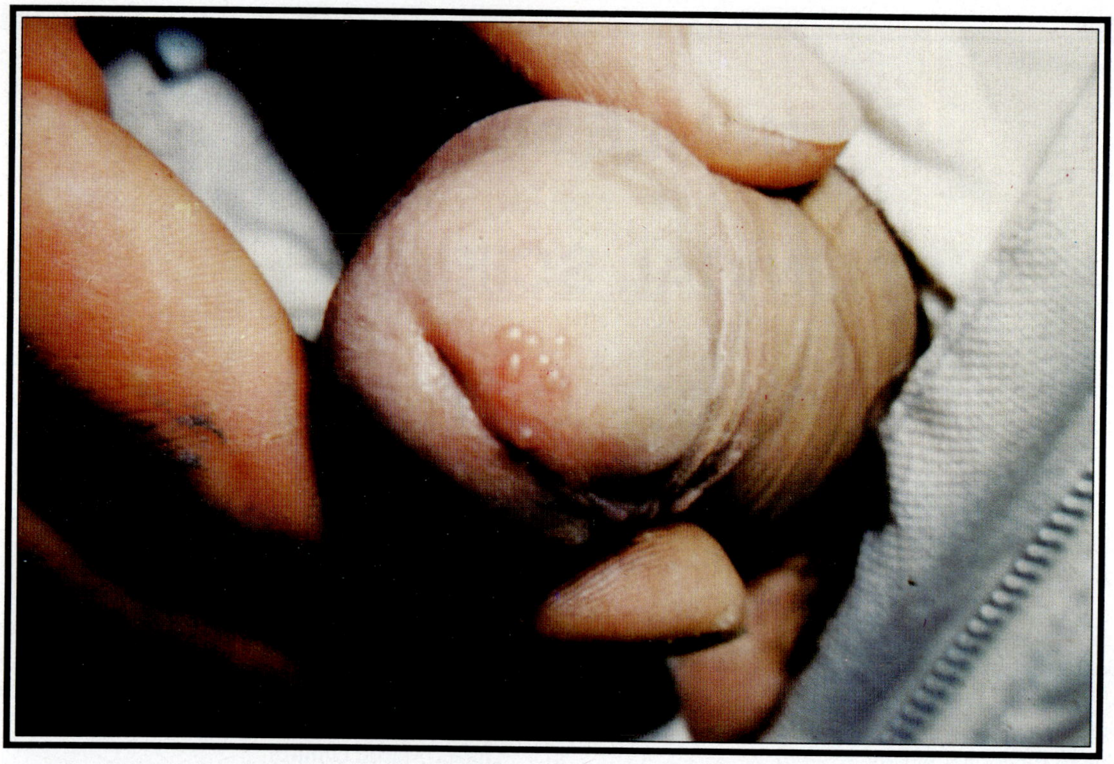

Figure C.9

Item 6-7

A 69-year-old white female is in the critical care unit after having severe chest pain. She has a history of hypertension, diabetes mellitus, hyperlipidemia and a myocardial infarct one year ago. In the critical care unit her BP is stable 120/70 mm Hg, pulse 90 bpm regular and her lungs are clear. Heart sounds reveal a S4. EKG during admission showed elevation of ST segment in the anterior wall. During the course of the night, the monitor shows the following abnormal rhythm (see figure C.10).

6. The EKG shows:

a) atrial fibrillation
b) ventricular tachycardia
c) idioventricular tachycardia
d) junctional tachycardia
e) supraventricular tachycardia

7. The most appropriate intervention at this time is:

a) lidocaine i.v.
b) DC cardioversion
c) verapamil i.v.
d) beta adrenergic blocking agents i.v.
e) amiodarone p.o.

8. Which of the following is NOT a consequence of the methylxanthines administration?

a) Decrease in fatigue and increase in mental alertness
b) Stimulation of HCl secretion from the gastric mucosa
c) Increment in heart rate and cardiac output
d) Strong antidiuretic action by stimulation of ADH release
e) Bronchodilation

9. The following conditions in a patient undergoing a surgical procedure may suggest the diagnosis of myxedema, EXCEPT:

a) acute hypotension
b) severe CO_2 retention
c) failure to awake promptly from anesthesia
d) hypothermia
e) hyperreflexia

Figure C.10

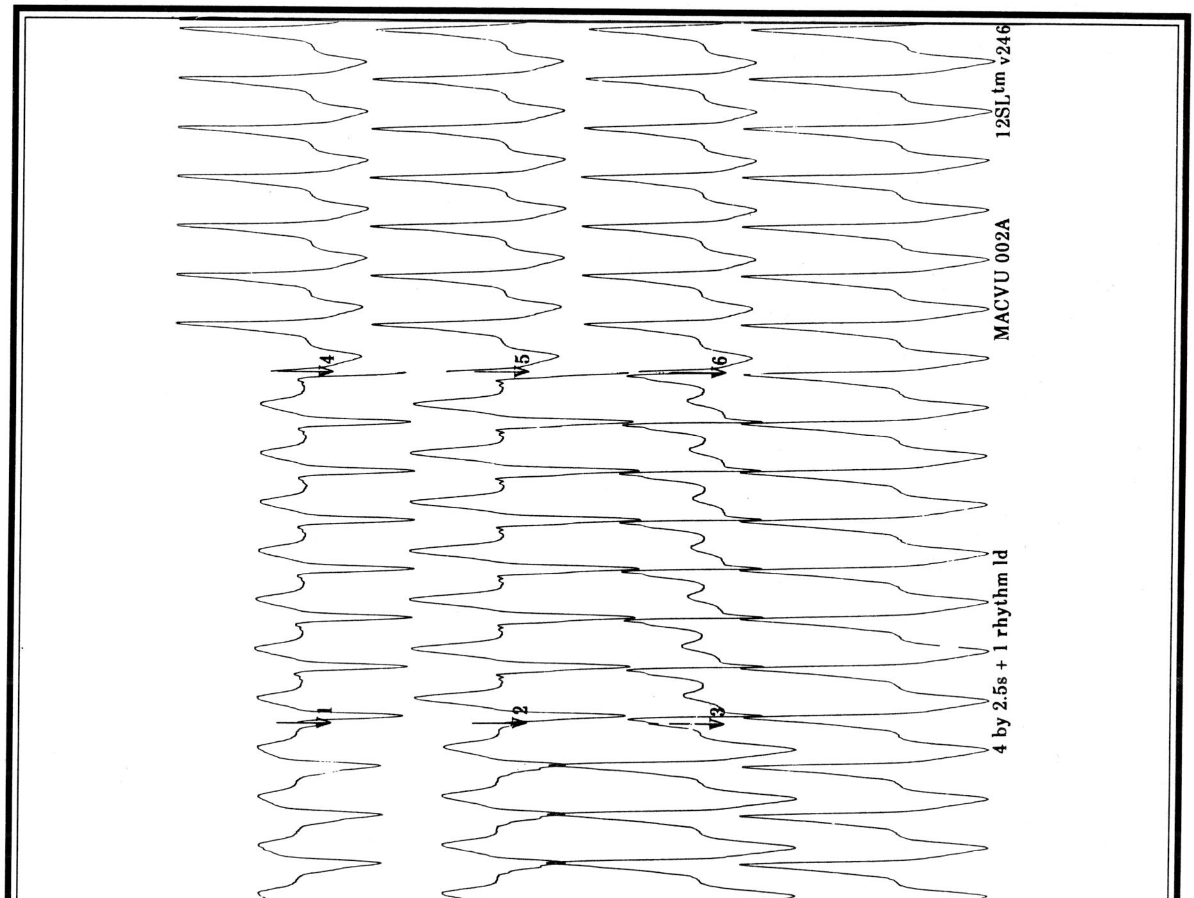
I
II
III
aVR
aVL
aVF
V1
V2
V3
V4
V5
V6
40 Hz
25.0 mm/s
10.0 mm/mV
4 by 2.5s + 1 rhythm ld
MACVU 002A
12SLtm v246

Items 10-12

A 60-year-old white male, farmer complains of low back pain during the last 3 months. An extensive testing was performed included MRI of the spine. No abnormalities were found, but he complains that the pain is getting worse. He feels exhausted and very sick. He says «I'm going' downhill, Doc! This back has upset everything. I just can't....function. I can't get my work done. It's just taken away all my power. I haven't slept the whole night in weeks...» The patient's lip quivers, but he recovers quickly, swallows hard, sets his shoulders and says, «since my wife died 8 months ago, I'm not worth a damn like this, Doc... .» He is constantly thinking of dying.

10. This patient should be treated with:

a) analgesic non-narcotic
b) morphine
c) non-steroidal anti-inflammatory agents
d) anti-depressive agents
e) hormone replacement

11. The diagnostic work up may include:

a) CT scan of chest and abdomen
b) myelography
c) bone scan
d) calcium and parathohormone serum levels
e) a trial of antidepressive medications

12. True statements regarding this patient's disease are the following, EXCEPT:

a) empathetic reassurance is usually worthwhile when the probability of serious disease is small
b) this disease is remarkable often encountered by primary care practicioners
c) this disease process is compatible with a major psychiatric disability
d) the probability of suicidal attempt in this patient is high
e) the sleep disorder in this patient most likely involves early morning awakening and/or difficulty falling asleep.

13. The following are common conditions or factors that may exacerbate or precipitate congestive heart failure, EXCEPT:

a) fluctuations in heart rate
b) increase in blood pressure
c) excess of blood volume
d) severe hypoxemia
e) the use of vasopressor agents

14. Which of the following statements regarding diabetes mellitus (DM) is INCORRECT?

a) DM type I is associated with a deficient insulin secretion
b) Patients with DM type I often present an immune-mediated destruction of the pancreatic beta cells
c) DM type II is most likely to cause ketoacidosis if exogenous insulin is withheld
d) The percentage of glycosilated hemoglobin in blood reflects the blood glucose levels over a period of 2-3 months before the current measurement
e) Obesity is characterized by decreased number or affinity of insulin receptors

Items 15-17

A 24-year-old white female patient presents with a low-grade fever (101°F), pleuritic chest pain, and dry nonproductive cough. She complains of muscle aches and severe headache. Her illness has evolved gradually over one weak. The sputum gram stain reveals rare neutrophils and no bacteria. She does not have history of HIV or other immunosuppressive disease. A chest-x-ray was obtained (see figure C.11).

15. Which of the following diagnostic tests can be performed in order to make the diagnosis of this disease?

a) CT scan of the chest
b) Cardiac isoenzymes
c) Cold agglutination serology
d) Bronchoscopy and bronchoalveolar lavage
e) DLCO

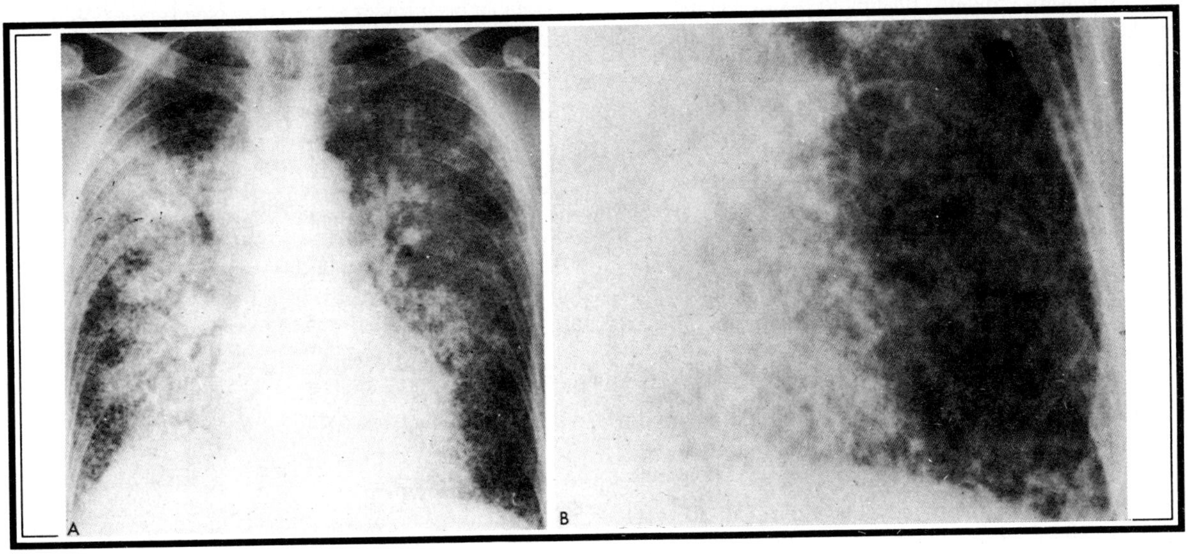

Figure C.11

16. The most remarkable finding in the chest-x-ray is:

a) pleural effusion
b) fibrocaseating tuberculosis
c) lobar consolidation
d) interstitial infiltrate
e) atelectasia of left lobe

17. You may treat this patient with:

a) erythromycin
b) at least four antibiotics for 6 months
c) amoxicillin/clavulanate
d) co-trimoxazole (TMP/SMX)
e) none of the above

18. A stiff neck or meningismus associated with headache is usually seen in:

a) deep neck abscesses
b) cervical osteomyelitis
c) brain abscess
d) complicated sinusitis
e) all of the above

19. Which of the following features is LEAST likely to be seen in classic migraine?

a) Visual or neurological prodrome
b) Throbbing, pulsatile headache
c) Bilateral headache
d) Photophobia
e) Nighttime headache

Items 20-22

A 50-year-old white male is admitted for chest pain and syncope. Blood pressure is 140/90 mm Hg and the pulse is slow rising-slow falling (anacrotic). The apex beat is displaced laterally. The second heart sound is diminished with reversed splitting. A rough ejection mid-systolic murmur is auscultable in the second right intercostal space.

20. Which of the following is the most likely cardiac valvular disease in this patient?

a) Mitral stenosis
b) Mitral regurgitation
c) Aortic stenosis
d) Aortic regurgitation
e) Atrial-septal defect

21. Which of the following conditions or complications is UNLIKELY to be present in patients with this critical valvular disease?

a) Left ventricular hypertrophy
b) Sudden death
c) Aortic valve endocarditis
d) peak systolic gradient < 10 mm Hg
e) Congestive heart failure

22. The following are considered poor prognosis markers for this disease, EXCEPT

a) syncope
b) angina pectoris
c) dyspnea
d) congestive heart failure
e) age below 50

23. The management of non-insulin dependent diabetic patients treated with oral agents in the preoperative stage include the following, EXCEPT:

a) if the serum glucose level is below 250 mg/dl on the morning of the surgery, sulfonylureas should be withheld
b) if the fasting glucose level is above 250-300 mg/dl, 5 units of regular insulin can be added to each liter of 5% glucose solution being given in infusion at 100 mL/h
c) the goal is to maintain glucose levels between 100 and 200 mg/dl before and after the surgical procedure
d) if blood sugar is 100-250 mg/dl the morning of the surgery, oral hypoglycemic agents should be given and additional doses of regular insulin should be injected before surgery to prevent the stress hyperglycemia
e) non-insulin dependent diabetic patients produce and secrete enough insulin to prevent ketoacidosis

Items 24-25

A 28-year-old white female presents with fever (102°F), sore throat, and general malaise. She has no significant previous medical history. She is taking no medications and she uses mechanical devices for contraception. Her physical examination is unremarkable except for pharyngeal erythema with normal tonsil size and the presence of several small anterior cervical lymphadenopathy. Five days after her initial symptoms, painful lesions in both lower extremities (see figure C.12) were noted.

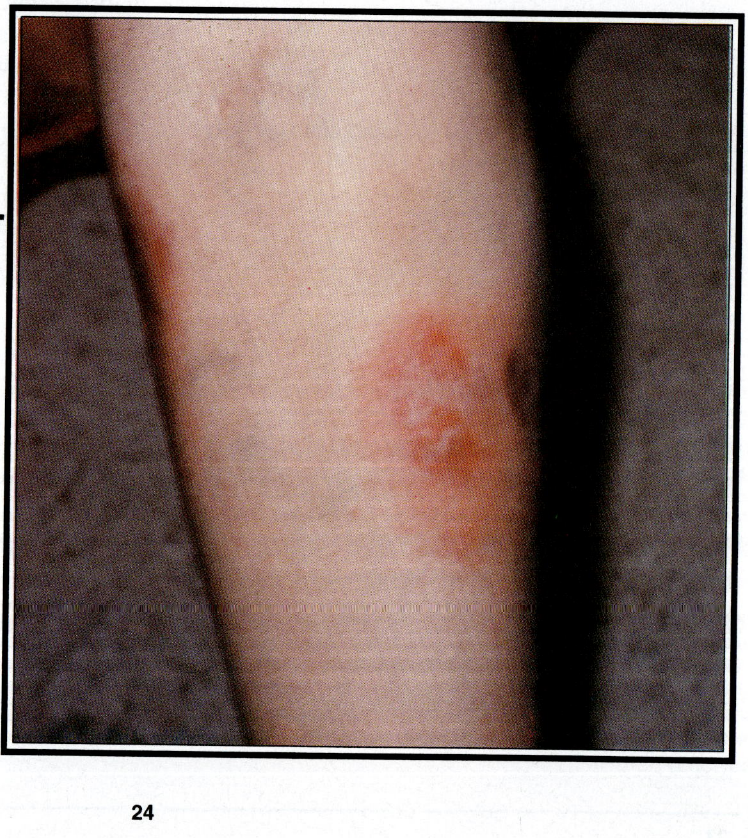

Figure C.12

24. The skin lesions are most likely:

a) erythema migrans
b) eczematous dermatitis
c) atopic dermatitis
d) psoriasis
e) erythema nodosum

25. The most common cause of these lesions are the following, EXCEPT:

a) streptococcus infection
b) tuberculosis
c) sarcoidosis
d) oral contraceptives
e) aspirin

Items 26-29

Match the clinical presentations of patients with peptic ulcer disease (PUD) with the most likely complication.

a) Perforation
b) Dumping syndrome
c) Gastric outlet obstruction
d) Gastrointestinal bleeding
e) None of the above

26. It occurs most frequently in those ulcers situated close to the pyloric channel.

27. It is most common along the anterior portion of the duodenal bulb.

28. It may result from a rapid gastric emptying of a large osmotic load.

29. A plain upright radiograph of the abdomen may show the presence of free air under the diaphragm.

30. In elderly patients that require surgical intervention, it should be considered:

a) a careful monitoring of intake, output, body weight, serum electrolytes and central venous pressure
b) they are more tolerant and less sensitive to the administration of anxiolytic medications
c) the administration of intravenous fluids may precipitate a circulatory volume overload
d) preanesthetic medications should be limited to atropine or scopolamine
e) sedative and hypnotic drugs may cause restlessness, mental confusion and uncooperative behavior

Items 31-36

Match the laboratory tests for hemostasis with their clinical indications and findings.

a) Prothrombin time
b) Template bleeding time
c) Activated partial thromboplastin time
d) Ristocetin-induced platelet agglutination
e) Factor IX concentration

31. It is prolonged in thrombocytopenia (<100,000/ uL), qualitative platelet disorders and vascular disorders.

32. Clotting time measured after addition of tissue factor and phospholipids to recalcified plasma.

33. This test depends on the intact intrinsic and common coagulation pathways.

34. It may be abnormal in patients treated with aspirin-containing medications.

35. Prolongation of this test occurs in deficiencies of factor VII, V, X, prothrombin or fibrinogen (<100 mg/ dl).

36. Assesses the presence of plasmatic von Willebrand factor.

Items 37-39

A 32-year-old white female complains of arthralgias in her hands and knees with fever, malaise, weight loss and nycturia. She noticed a facial rash (see figure C.13) after sun exposure that persists for months. The physical examination shows BP 180/110 mm Hg, pericardial rub and arthritis in both knees with (+) edema in the lower extremities.

37 Which is the most likely diagnoses in this patient?

a) Systemic lupus erythematosus
b) Infectious arthritis
c) Psoriatic arthritis
d) Still's disease
e) Rheumatoid arthritis

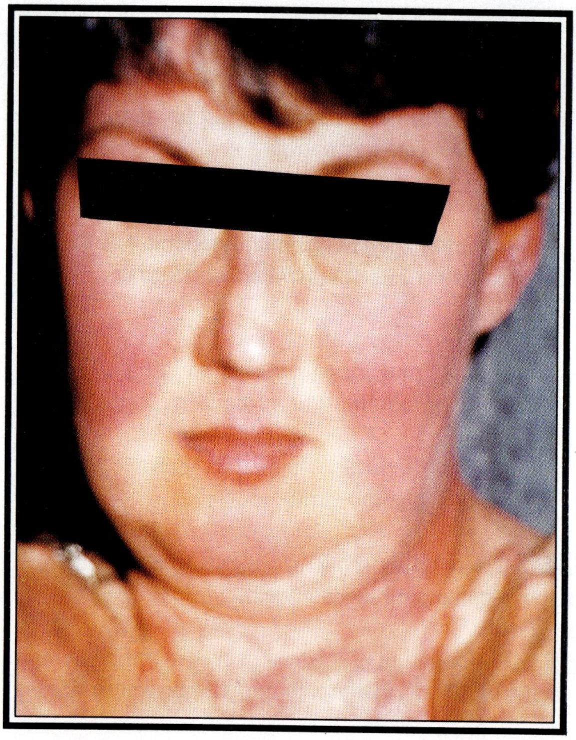

Figure C.13

38. Which of the following is LEAST likely a complication in the course of this disease?

a) Pneumonitis
b) Infertility
c) Myocarditis
d) Leukopenia
e) Chronic leukemia

39. Which of the following is NOT an appropriate therapeutic intervention in the course of the disease?

a) Non-steroidal antiinflammatory drugs
b) Hydroxychloroquine in the subacute cutaneous lupus
c) Glucocorticoids in life-threatening disease
d) Cyclophosphamide in patients refractory to non-steroidal antiinflammatory drugs
e) Kidney transplantation

40. The following conditions are responsible for a delayed wound healing, EXCEPT:

a) protein depletion
b) ascorbic acid deficiency
c) marked dehydration
d) severe anemia
e) vitamin K deficiency

Items 41-44

A 47-year-old alcoholic patient is admitted to the intensive care unit, confuse with hypotension refractory to i.v. fluid and oliguria. His physical examination reveals jaundice, BP is 70/40 mm, temperature 103°F, pulse 134 bpm, tachypnea (44 respirations/minute), poor peripheral perfusion, with copious crackles in both lungs. Heart presents tachycardia with normal sounds. Abdomen is distended with ascites and no bowel sounds. Chest-x-ray was obtained (see figure C.14).

41. Which is the most likely cause of this picture?

a) Uncontrolled sepsis
b) Gastrointestinal bleeding
c) Hypovolemic shock
d) Laenec's cirrhosis
e) An autoimmune disease

42. The chest roentgenogram shows:

a) tension pneumothorax
b) ARDS
c) lobar pneumonia
d) milliar tuberculosis
e) bilateral pleural effusion

43. Which of the following is NOT an appropriate intervention at this time?

a) Swan-ganz catheter placement
b) Intravenous fluid and vasopressor drugs
c) Oxygenation and mechanical ventilatory support
d) Heparin in bolus followed by infusion
e) Diuretics i.v.

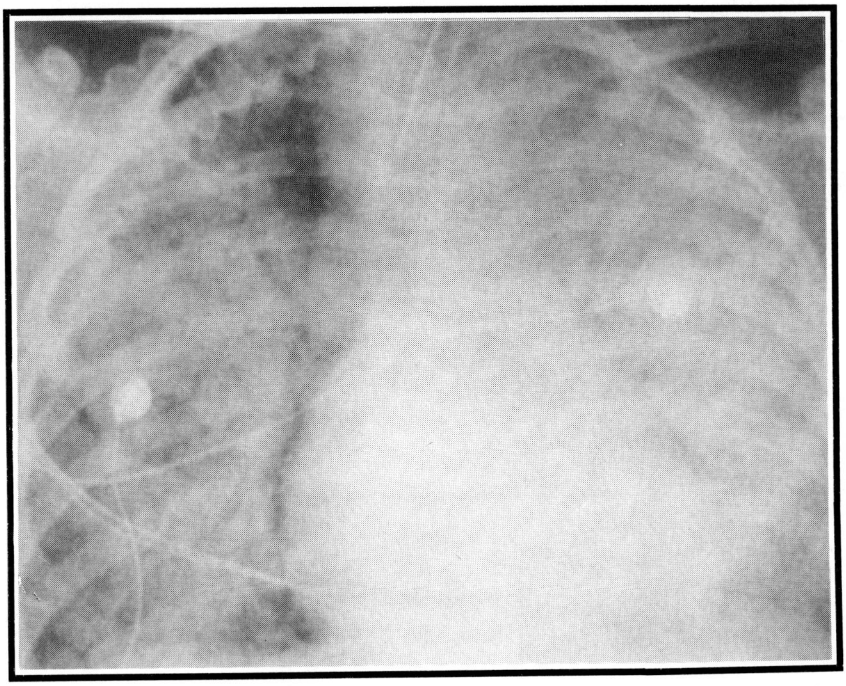

Figure C.14

44. Which of the following statements regarding this clinical picture is INCORRECT?

a) Infectious agents in this patient are usually gram negative aerobic bacteria
b) In this setting the mortality is up to 60- 90%
c) Poor organ perfusion and organ ischemia is usually seen in early and later stages of this condition
d) Dobutamine is used for its direct vasoconstrictor effect
e) Systemic vascular resistance is decreased in this patient

45. Burkitt's lymphoma:

a) is associated with HIV virus infection
b) presents abundance in Reed-Sternberg cells with lymphocytic repletion
c) is a primary extralymphatic african tumor arising from jawbones
d) is most frequent in Japan
e) is a good prognosis hematologic tumor

46. A 28-year-old patient complains of fever (40°C), purpura and bleeding of the gums. Peripheral blood analysis shows 75,000 cell/mm3 with 90% blasts. The most probable diagnosis is:

a) chronic leukemia
b) acute leukemia
c) miliary tuberculosis
d) acquired immunodeficiency syndrome
e) multiple myeloma

Item 47

A 19-year-old man is found to have an acute leukemia. He received two cycles of chemotherapy in the course of one month. During the hospital course he has a spiking temperature of 40°C when his white blood cell count was 800/uL. Which of the following statements regarding this clinical condition is INCORRECT?

Figure C.15

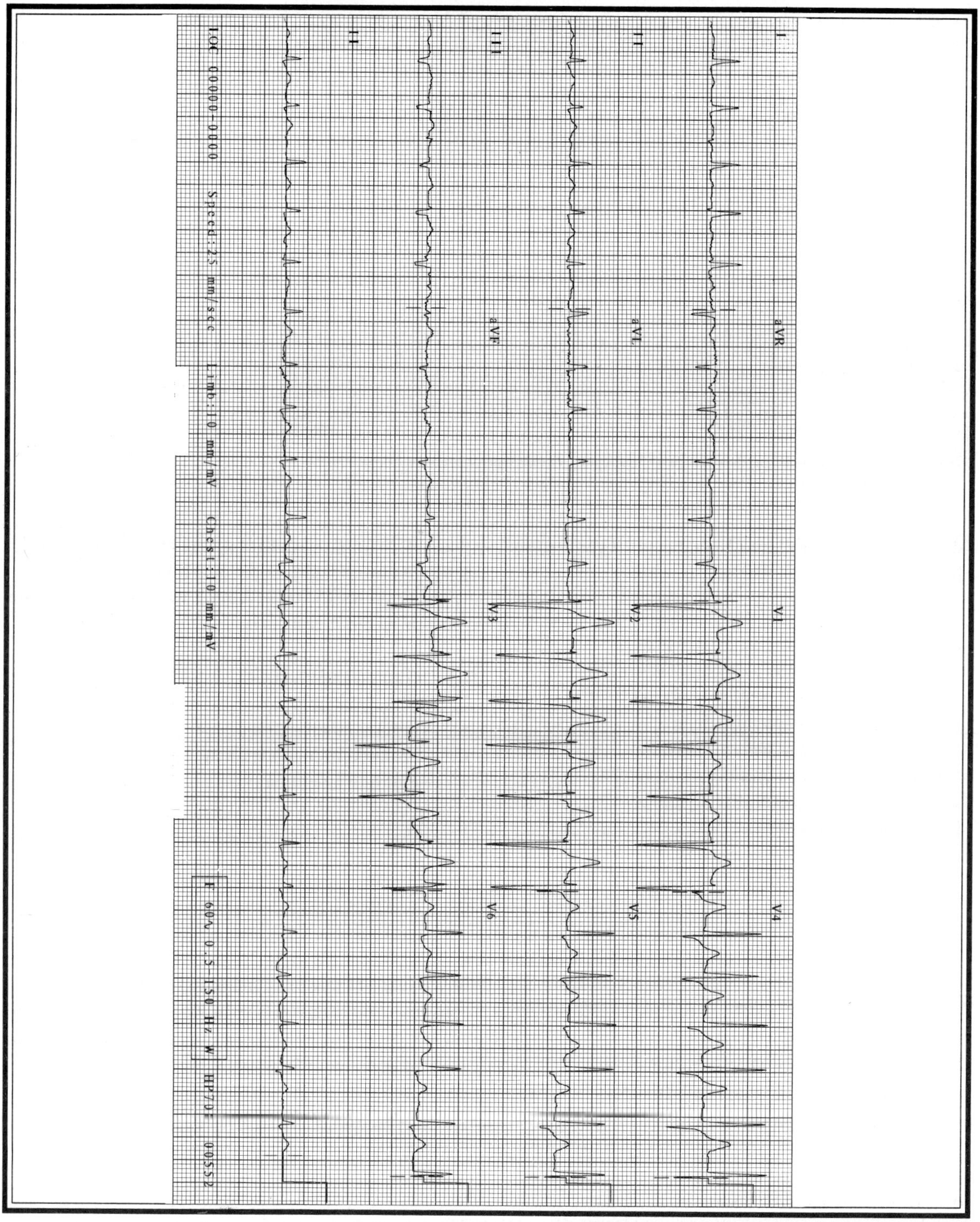
I
aVR
V1
V4
II
aVL
V2
V5
III
aVF
V3
V6
II
LOC 00000-0000 Speed:25 mm/sec Limb:10 mm/mV Chest:10 mm/mV
F 60~ 0.5-150 Hz W
00552

a) Normal chest-x-ray would not rule-out pneumonia
b) Infection is the most common cause of mortality in these patients
c) Gram positive coccus are responsible for most pneumonias and bacteremias
d) A cephalosporin plus an aminoglycoside is a commonly used regimen to treat this fever
e) Chemotherapy should be stopped until infection is controlled and white count improves

Item 48-49

A 62-year-old black female is seen for recurrent palpitations. She is hypertensive, treated with hydrochlorothiazide for the last 4 years. Her physical examination is unremarkable except for tachycardia and irregular pulse (140 bpm). Blood pressure is 160/ 90 mm Hg. EKG is shown in the figure C.15.

48. The EKG shows:

a) atrial fibrillation
b) atrial flutter
c) junctional tachycardia
d) wondering pacemaker
e) ventricular tachycardia

49. The MOST appropriate treatment at this time is:

a) digital
b) intravenous lidocaine
c) DC cardioversion
d) diltiazem
e) per oral beta blocker agents

50. Which of the following is NOT a common feature of the Zollinger-Ellison syndrome?

a) Diarrhea
b) Refractory peptic ulcer disease
c) Lack of response to secretin stimulation test
d) Basal gastric acid hypersecretion
e) Hypertrophy of the gastric mucosa

51. The most sensitive test to determine body iron stores is:

a) plasmatic TIBC level
b) plasmatic ferritin level
c) bone marrow iron stain
d) red cell hemoglobin level
e) electrophoresis of serum proteins

52. Which of the following antibodies is most specific in the diagnoses of primary biliary cirrhosis?

a) Anti-DNA
b) Anti-mitochondrial
c) Anti-myeloperoxidase
d) Anti-cytoplasmatic neutrophil antibody
e) Anti-Sm

53. The following are the most common clinical findings in hematochromatosis, EXCEPT:

a) diabetes mellitus
b) hepatocellular carcinoma
c) pulmonary fibrosis
d) testicular atrophy
e) change in skin pigmentation

Items 54-56

A 45-year-old patient is admitted with pallor of the skin and mucous membranes, increase in pulse rate, palpitations, dizziness, and fatigue. He vomited twice the day of admission and he complains of severe left upper quadrant pain. He is a heavy drinker and he had a car accident 3 days ago with no medical evaluation.

54. Which of the following conditions must be suspected in this patient?

a) An acute myocardial infarct
b) A spleen rupture with severe anemia
c) An acute gastritis
d) A perforated peptic ulcer
e) None of the above

55. Which of the following is the most useful and appropriate diagnostic test?

a) EKG
b) Upper gastrointestinal endoscopy
c) Peritoneal lavage
d) Thallium stress test
e) Endoscopy

56. What is the most important therapeutic approach in this case?

a) Medical treatment
b) Transfusion and splenectomy
c) Surgical repair of the ulcer
d) Anti-angina medicines
e) Infusion of sclerosing agents

57. Which of the following statements regarding sickle cell anemia is INCORRECT?

a) This disorder results from a defect in hemoglobin structure
b) Traits occur in the heterozygous state along with normal adult hemoglobin in asymptomatic individuals
c) Antibodies, usually IgG class, are directed against red cells causing hemolysis
d) The abnormality consists of a single amino acid substitution in the beta-chain.
e) At low pH and with decreased oxygen tension, HbS precipitates

58. Which of the following characteristics of the colon and rectum carcinoma is INCORRECT?

a) Carcinoma of the colon and the rectum continues to be the most common cancer of the GI tract
b) It is the third most common cause of cancer in men, preceded only by cancer of lung and prostate
c) Changes in bowel habits and rectal bleeding may occur first
d) Prognosis does not correlate with Duke's classification
e) Obstruction is more common in carcinoma of the left colon

Items 59-60

A 62-year-old white male is admitted to the hospital after the onset of fever (101°F), malaise and vesicular exanthem in various stages of evolution (see figure C.16). He denied any previous medical diseases, travel outside of town, or weight loss. His physical examination is unremarkable except for the rash mostly seen in his trunk and upper extremities.

59. The most likely disease is:

a) Herpes simplex
b) Varicella
c) Rocky mountain fever
d) Cytomegalovirus
e) Measles

60. The following are common complications of this clinical presentation, EXCEPT:

a) pneumonia
b) Guillain Barre syndrome
c) encephalitis
d) malignancy
e) bacterial superinfection of the skin

FIgure C.16

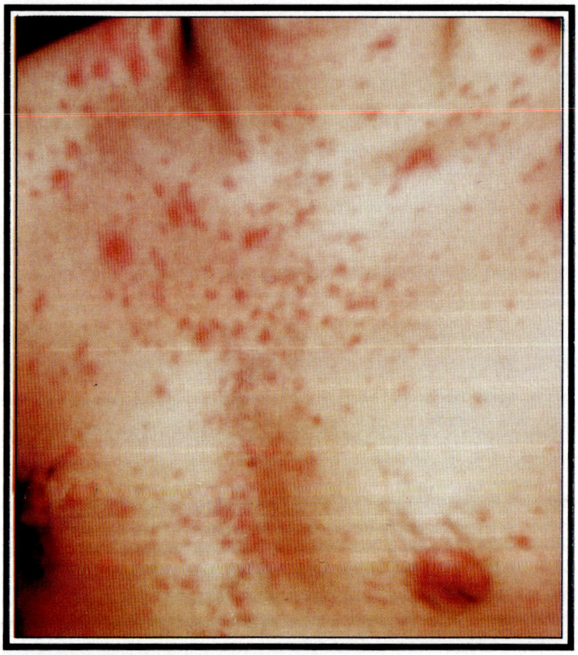

61. Which of the following disorders is NOT associated with high output heart failure?

a) Thyrotoxicosis
b) Cardiac tamponade
c) Beri-beri
d) Systemic arteriovenous fistula
e) Vascular shunts

62. Which of the following statements regarding the physiologic control of the eating behavior is INCORRECT?

a) Thalamus controls hunger and eating
b) Lesions of the lateral hypothalamus cause anorexia
c) Electrical stimulation of the lateral hypothalamus can produce immediate vigorous eating behavior
d) Lesions in the ventromedial hypothalamus produce extreme obesity

Items 63-64

A 59-year-old white male is having an elective prostatectomy. He has a history of lung disease due to asbestos exposure for 30 years. He is not taking any medications and his physical examination is unremarkable except for fine crackles scattered in both lungs. His pre-operative evaluation reveals:

pH	7.42	
pO2	68	mm Hg
pCO2	37	mm Hg
Bicarbonate	24	mEq/l
Tidal Volume	400	cc
Min Volume	6,000	cc
FVE1	3,000	cc
Vital Capacity	3,200	cc
FVE1/VC	94	%
Residual volume	80	%
DLCO	70	%

63. Which is the most likely pulmonary functional abnormality or disease?

a) COPD with moderate obstructive airway disease
b) COPD with severe obstructive airway disease
c) Restrictive lung disease
d) asthma
e) None of the above

64. This patient:

a) may require mechanical ventilation after surgery
b) should quit smoking at least four days before surgery
c) should receive solumedrol intravenous 2 hours before surgery
d) requires theophylline i.v. during the surgical procedure
e) none of the above

65. Xanthomas seen in a patient with chronic liver disease may suggest the diagnosis of:

a) hemochromatosis
b) hepatitis B
c) primary biliary cirrhosis
d) lupus hepatitis
e) drug-induced hepatitis

66. Which of the following is LEAST likely a complication seen in liver cirrhosis?

a) Portal hypertension and gastrointestinal hemorrhage
b) Portosystemic encephalopathy
c) Peptic ulcer disease
d) Ulcerative colitis
e) Esophageal varices

67. Which of the following is NOT a cause of severe splenomegaly?

a) Chronic myeloid leukemia
b) Visceral leishmaniasis
c) Bacterial endocarditis
d) Portal hypertension
e) Hydatid disease

68. Urgency, precipitancy and frequency of micturition are common symptoms in:

a) nervous system disease such as multiple sclerosis
b) bladder tumor
c) urinary infection
d) cystitis
e) all of the above

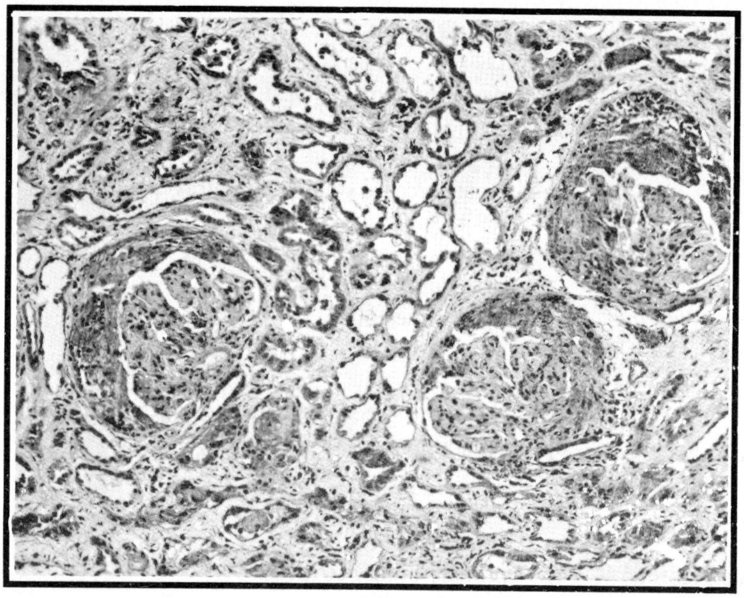

Figure C.17

URINE		
Specific Gravity	1012	
Protein	3 (+)	
RBC	-	
WBC	2-3	/ hpf

Two days later, the serum creatinine rose to 10.7 mg/dL and the creatinine clearance came down to 8.4 ml/min.

Items 69-73

A 65-year-old man is admitted with a 4-day history of hematuria, chills, fever, and generalized aches. He has history of heavy smoking and alcohol abuse. He denies any other significant medical history and he is not taking any medications. BP is 160/80 mm Hg, temperature, 103°F. The rest of the physical examination is unremarkable except for mild edema in the lower extremities. One week after admission, oliguria developed and the patient gradually became anuric. A renal biopsy was performed (see figure C.17).

Laboratory analysis:

BLOOD		
Sodium	138	mEq/L
Potassium	4.3	mEq/L
Glucose	170	mg/dL
BUN	44	mg/dL
Creatinine	3.9	mg/dL
LDH	210	U/L
Serum protein	6.8	g/dL
Serum albumin	2.8	g/dL
WBC	9,600	cells/uL
Hemoglobin	13	mg/dl
Platelets	190,000	platelets/ul
Sedimentation rate	88	mm/hr
ASO titer	normal	
ANA titer	negative	

69. Which is the most likely diagnosis?

a) Lupus erythematous systemic
b) Alport's syndrome
c) Diffuse proliferative and exudative glomerulonephritis
d) Minimal changes glomerulonephritis
e) Idiopathic rapidly progressive glomerulonephritis

70. Light microscopy shows (see figure C.17):

a) glomeruli show florid epithelial crescents
b) tubules may show hyalin droplets and fatty changes
c) the capillary lumina are wide open
d) interstitium and blood vessels are free of inflammatory infiltrated
e) none of the above

71. Which of the following statements regarding this disease process is INCORRECT?

a) Nearly all patients are admitted in renal failure with azotemia, oliguria
b) Most cases follow beta hemolytic group A streptococcus infection
c) They develop irreversible renal failure
d) The ASO titer and serum complement are normal
e) Renal arteriogram shows normal-sized or enlarged kidneys strongly suggestive of a recent acute process

72. The treatment of choice is:

a) plasmapheresis
b) steroids
c) cyclophosphamide
d) bactrim
e) dialysis

73. The following are common diseases with similar clinical presentations, EXCEPT:

a) Goodpasture's syndrome
b) fulminant poststreptococcal glomerulonephritis
c) progressive anaphylactoid purpura
d) polyarteritis nodosa
e) drug-induced nephropathy

Items 74-75

Match the features of the following psychological stages of the dying patient.

a) Denial
b) Anger
c) Bargaining
d) Depression
e) None of the above

74. Emotional detachment and a relinquishing of social and family bonds and responsibilities.

75. Search for meaning in life and often by a return to religious institutions. This stage is marked by a belief that some magical power will intervene.

76. Which of the following is NOT an indication for tuberculin skin-testing?

a) Persons with signs and symptoms associated with chest-x-ray abnormalities
b) Recent contacts of persons known to have or suspected of having clinically active tuberculosis
c) Persons with HIV infection
d) Elderly that is being placed in a nursing home
e) General population screening

77. Physicians should be aware that the following signs and symptoms are most frequently associated with alcohol abuse and dependence, EXCEPT:

a) denial of a problem in the face of a clear dysfunction due to alcohol intake
b) concern with control of the alcohol abuse
c) family, work or school problems
d) conversion disorder
e) evidences of depression

78. All the following statements regarding opiates dependency are correct, EXCEPT:

a) patient complains of illnesses that require pain medication
b) use of multiple drugs prescribed by many physicians
c) a feeling on the part of the physician of being manipulated
d) treatment should include aversive therapy and isolation
e) patients are usually of young age

Figure C.18

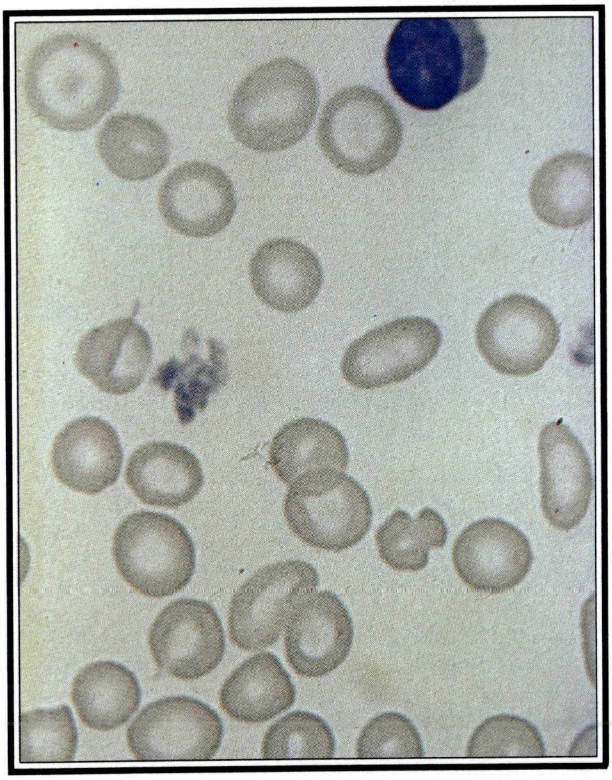

Figure C.19

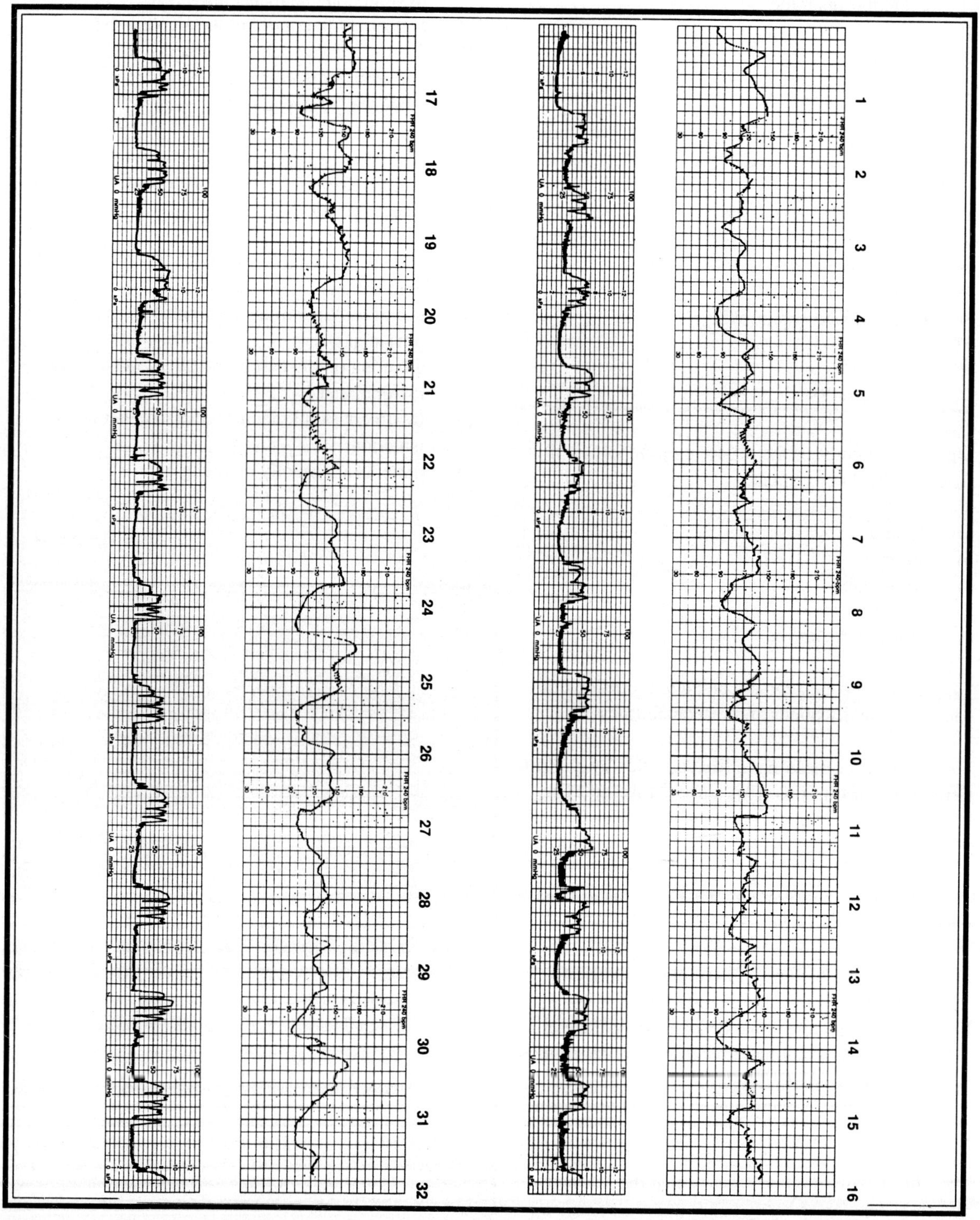

79. The following picture (see figure C.18) shows a peripheral blood smear of an alcoholic patient with anemia. According to the smear, the most likely cause of the anemia is:

a) vitamin C deficiency
b) vitamin B12 deficiency
c) iron deficiency
d) bone marrow toxicity
e) portal hypertension

Item 80

A 37-week-pregnant white female is admitted to the hospital after having symptoms of labor and severe abdominal pain with vaginal bleeding. A tracing of fetal heart rate and uterine contractions is obtained (see figure C.19).

80. The tracing shows:

a) that the fetus responds with constant accelerations
b) that the fetus does not respond to uterine contractions
c) that the baseline variability is extraordinarily high
d) that with each contraction the fetus responds with variable decelerations
e) that the majority of the variable decelerations are accompanied by ample overshoot patterns

Item 81

A 49-year-old white male with a history of chronic renal failure in a dialysis program three times a week, is admitted to the critical care unit for changes in mental status. He was in anasarca with oligoanuria. His BP 180/100 mm Hg, pulse 140 bpm regular. Jugulars were engorged and bilateral fine crackles were auscultated in both lungs. S3 heart sound was present in gallop cadency. Marked bilateral pedal edema was seen in both lower extremities. An admission EKG was normal. Next day blood samples for chemistry and an EKG were obtained (see figure C.20).

Laboratory analysis:

BLOOD		
Sodium	128	mEq/L
Potassium	7.0	mEq/L
Chloride	98	mEq/L
Calcium	8.2	mg /dL
Magnesium	1.4	mg/dL
Bicarbonate	10	mEq/L
Albumin	2.9	g/dL
Total Protein	5.1	g/dL
WBC	7,400	cells/uL
Hemoglobin	10	mg/dl
pH	7.25	
pO2	98	mm Hg
pCO2	23	mm Hg

81. The most likely explanation for the findings in the EKG is:

a) hypomagnesemia
b) hyponatremia
c) hyperkalemia
d) hypocalcemia
e) coronary insufficiency

82. Which of the following volume/pressure curves (cystograms) is the best representation of a genuine stress incontinence (GSI)?

a)
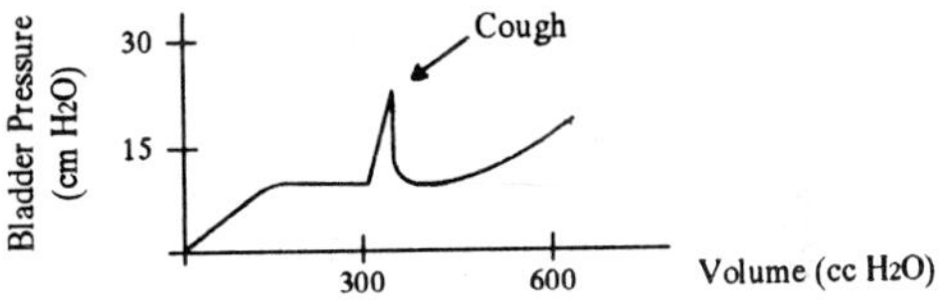

b)
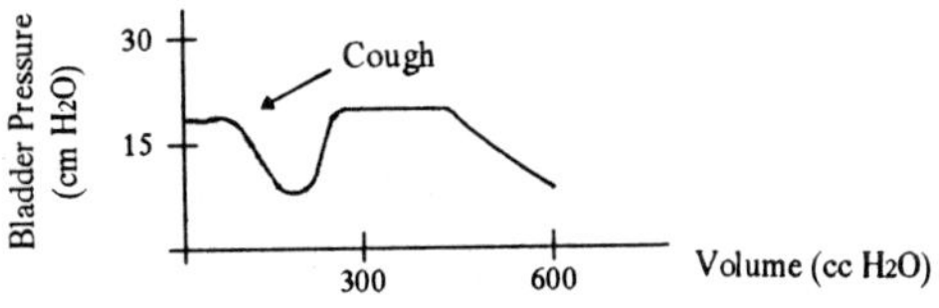

c)
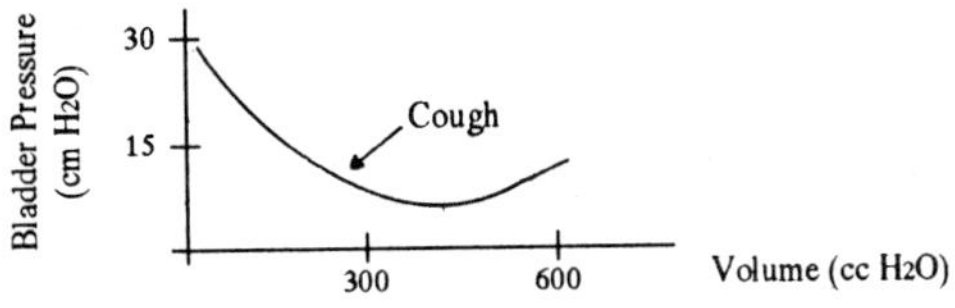

d)
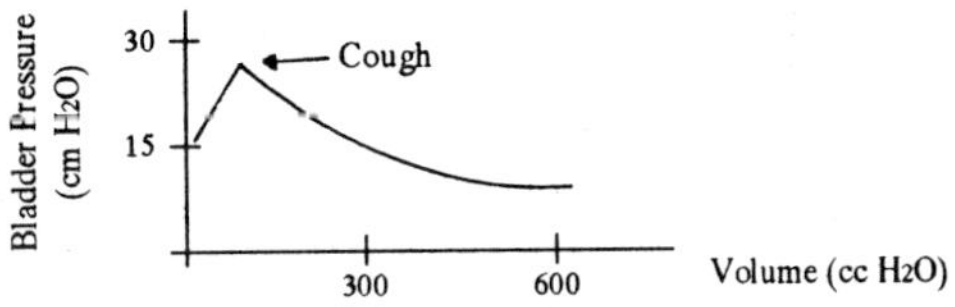

e) none of the above

Figure C.20

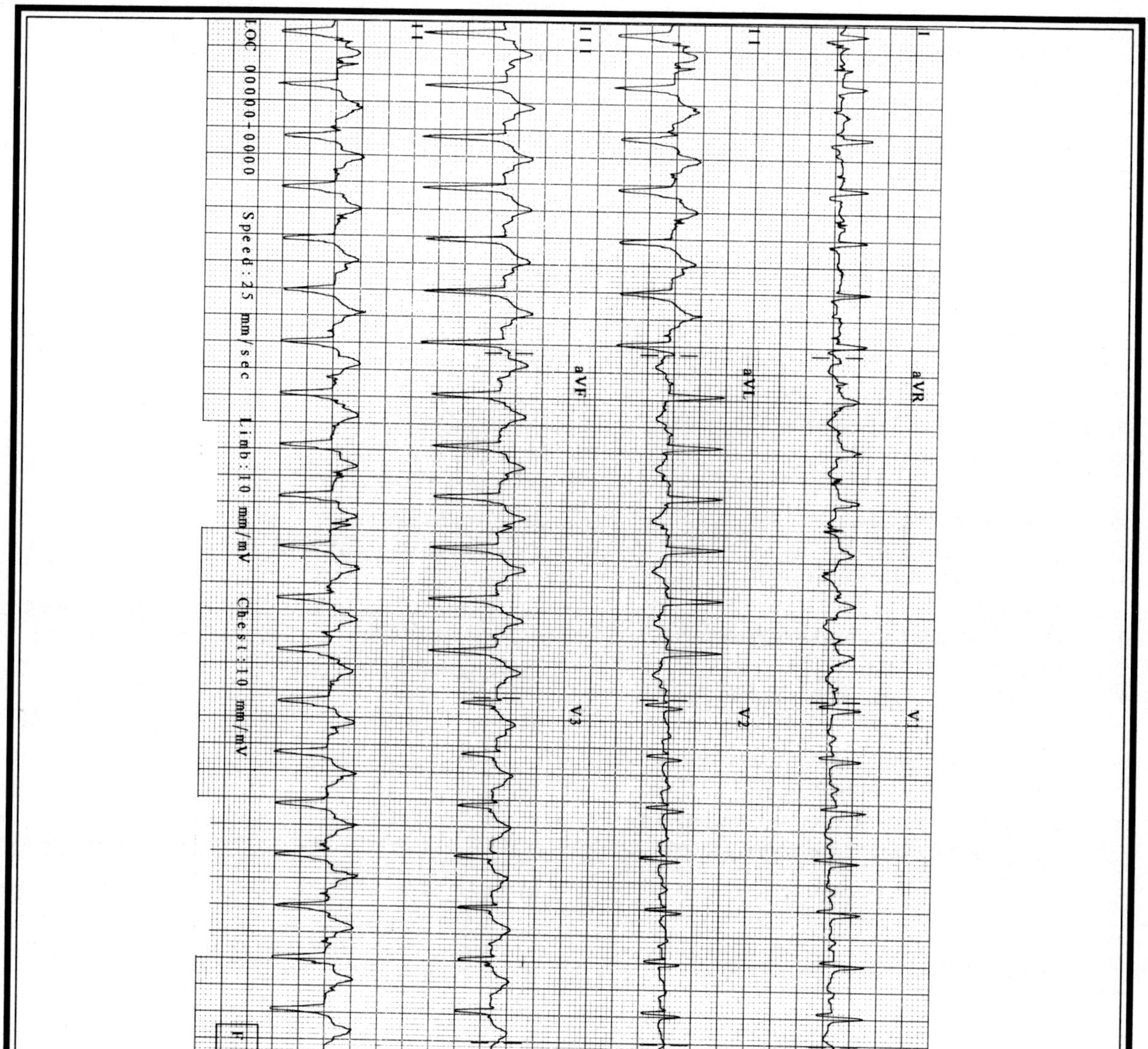
I
aVR
V1
V4
II
aVL
V2
V5
III
aVF
V3
V6
II
LOC 00000-0000
Speed: 25 mm/sec
Limb: 10 mm/mV
Chest: 10 mm/mV
F 60~ 0.5-100 Hz W
00543

Item 83-84

A 26-year-old white male is seen for severe chest pain. He is a heavy smoker and has a strong family history for coronary artery disease (father and mother had heart attacks before age 50). He has a previous history of alcohol and drug abuse. His physical examination reveals an obese hypotense (90/45 mm Hg) young male with tachycardia 118 bpm and breathing 26 times/minute. An early systolic II/VI murmur no modifiable with changes in positions or breathing is heard in mesocardium area. Lungs sounds are normal. Laboratory tests are unremarkable and drug screen in urine is pending. An admission EKG is shown in figure C.21.

83. The following possible conditions or diseases should be included in the differential diagnosis, EXCEPT:

a) hyperthyroidism
b) withdrawal from chronic exposure to nitroglycerin
c) vasospastic coronary disease
d) cocaine ingestion and overdoses
e) vasculitis

84. The EKG shows:

a) ischemia of lateral wall
b) inferior wall necrosis
c) right ventricular hypertrophy
d) inferior wall myocardial ischemia
e) acute pericarditis

Item 85

A 65-year-old white male is seen in a routine examination. He is asymptomatic and the physical examination is normal. An EKG was obtained (see figure C.22)

85. The abnormal finding in this EKG is:

a) ST segment elevation
b) left bundle branch block
c) right bundle branch block
d) second degree A-V block
e) old inferior myocardial infarct

Figure C.21

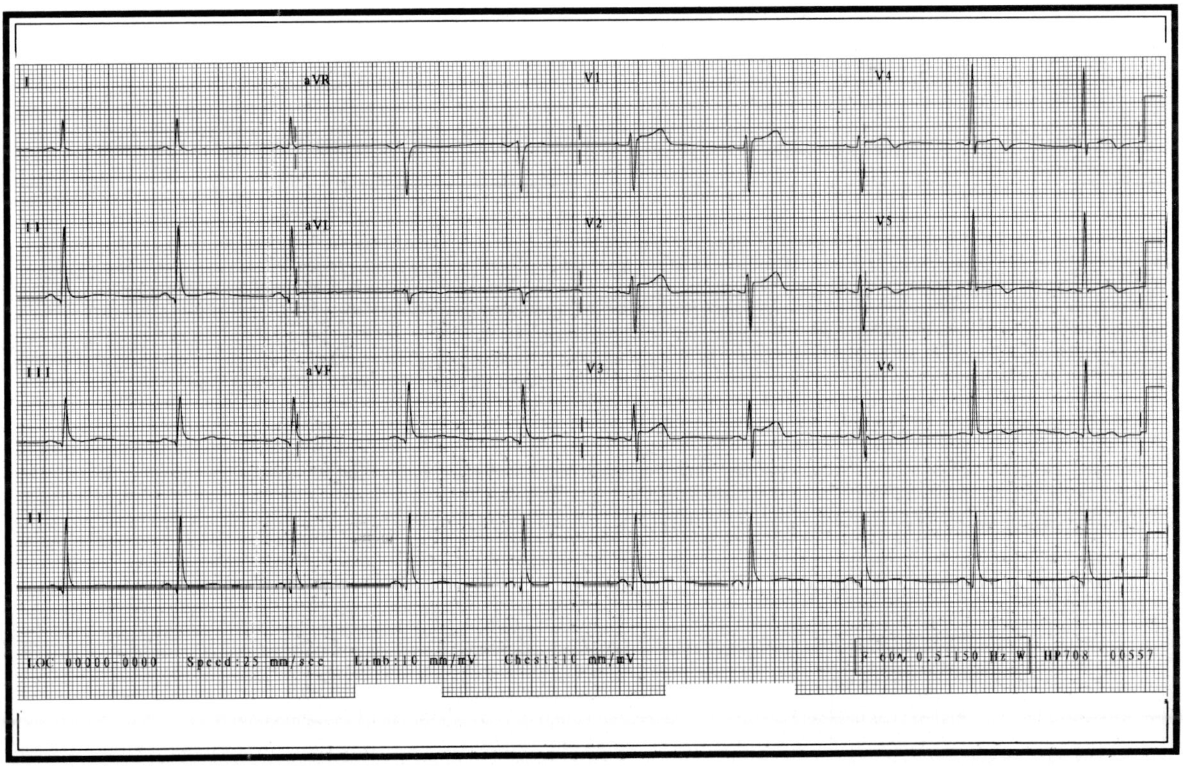

Figure C.22

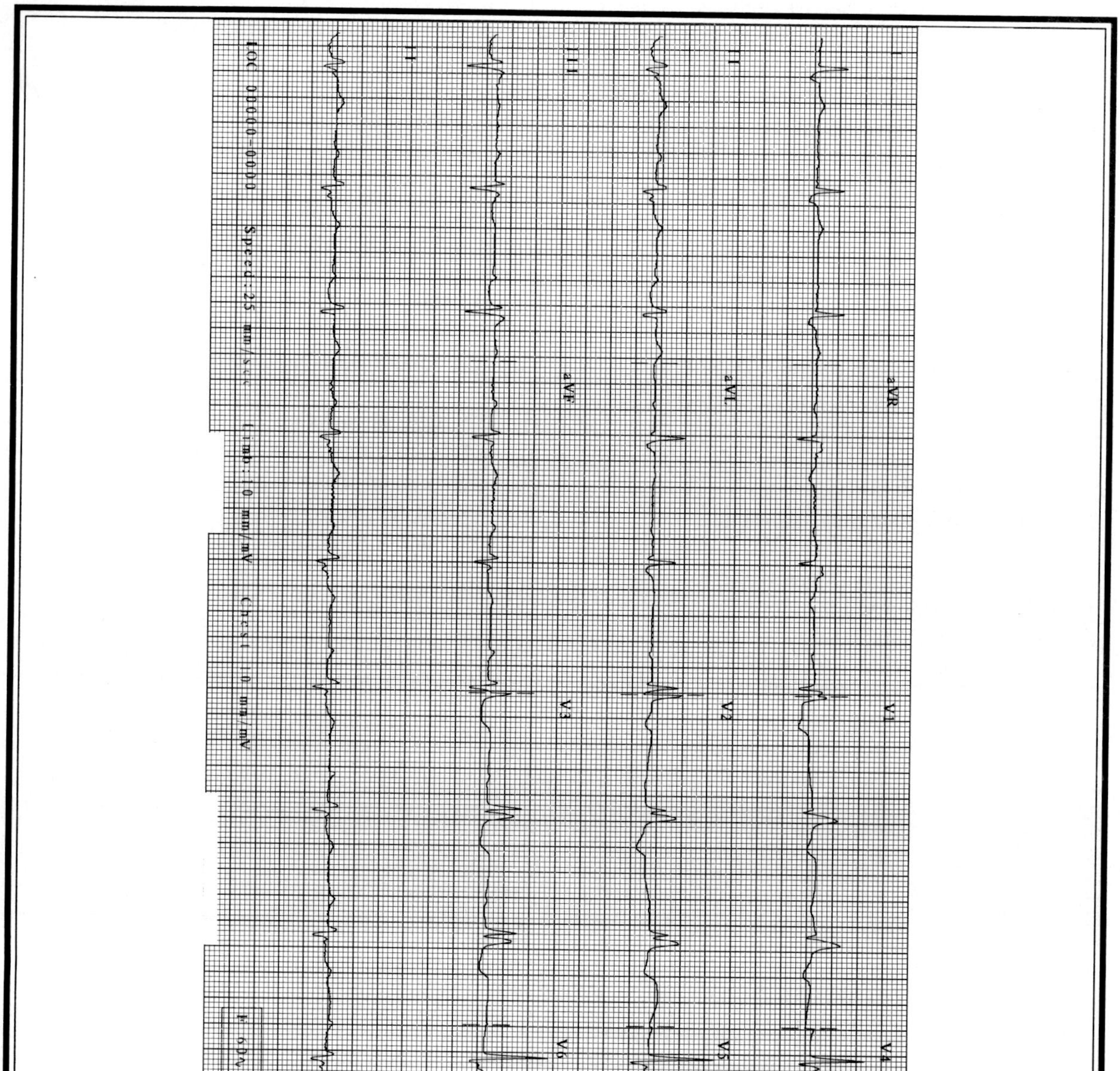
I
aVR
V1
V4
II
aVL
V2
V5
III
aVF
V3
V6
II
LOC 00000-0000 Speed:25 mm/sec Limb:10 mm/mV Chest:10 mm/mV
F 60~ 0.5-150 Hz W

86. In chronic pancreatitis:

a) usually does not present steatorrhea
b) is relapsing and infrequently it is associated with pancreatic exo and endocrine insufficiency
c) serum pancreatic isoamylase is usually elevated
d) to treat the pain in chronic pancreatitis, alcohol and narcotics should be withdrawn if possible
e) the pain is usually mild and exacerbated by eating

87. Which of the following statements regarding the treatment of esophageal varices is INCORRECT?

a) Endoscopy must be performed when the patient has become hemodynamically stable
b) Patients who do not respond to vasopressin treatment require immediate surgical treatment
c) Balloon tamponade with a Sengstaken-Blakemore tube can be used in the acute setting
d) Acute variceal hemorrhage may be controlled with a single injection of an sclerosing agent in 70 to 80% of patients
e) About half of patients treated by injection sclerotherapy will rebleed at some time

88. Which of the following statements regarding the diet and the serum lipoproteins is CORRECT?

a) Monounsaturated fat (approximately 15% of calories) and polyunsaturated fats (approximately 7% of calories) do not elevate LDL cholesterol
b) The important elements of the diet that primarily affect LDL cholesterol levels are saturated fat, cholesterol, caloric balance, and soluble fiber
c) An overabundance of calories will increase the triglyceride synthesis
d) Current guidelines for dietary modification to reduce cholesterol recommend reduction of saturated fat to less than 10% of calorics and cholesterol to less than 300 mg/day
e) Dietary cholesterol increases the number of LDL receptors in the liver and decrease in LDL concentrations

Items 89-91

An 60-year-old white female presents with fever, dysuria, frequency, urgency and dark urine for the last 4 days. She had a similar episode two years ago. She has non-insulin dependent diabetes mellitus and arterial hypertension treated with diabeta and nifedipine. On examination she is febrile (38oC), BP 120/80 mm Hg, pulse 110 bpm. Her abdomen is mildly distended with some tenderness in the low abdomen. Bladder is palpable.

Laboratory analysis:

BLOOD

Hb:	12	g/dl
MCV:	101	fl
WBC:	14 x 10^9	/l
Platelets:	170 x 10^9	/l
Sodium:	140	mEq/L
Potassium:	4.3	mEq/L
Chloride:	100	mEq/L
Urea:	18	mg/dL
Creatinine:	0.9	mg/dL
Bilirubin:	2.8	mg/dL
Albumin:	4.4	mg/dL
Total protein:	7.5	mg/dL

URINE

Urinalysis: protein +++; red cells++, bile++; urobilinogen++, WBC 50/field.

89. What is the MOST likely diagnosis?

a) Pelvic inflammatory disease
b) Nephrolithiasis
c) Ulcerative colitis
d) Lower urinary tract infection
e) Upper urinary tract infection

90. Which of the following statements regarding this disease is INCORRECT?

a) Urine collection under aseptic techniques often presents more than 103 bacteria/ml
b) Recurrent UTI may be associated with sexual activity
c) It usually occurs in women
d) Infections in men younger than 50 years of age are uncommon and suggest anatomic or functional abnormalities of the genitourinary tract
e) Chronic UTI is usually related to bladder instrumentation or catheterization

91. Which of the following treatments is the most appropriate in this patient?

a) Ciprofloxacine per oral
b) Erythromycin per oral
c) TMP/SMZ per oral
d) Folley catheter placement with continuous irrigation
e) None of the above

Items 92-95

A 35-year-old white male is admitted to the hospital for weight loss, general malaise, weakness cough and hemoptysis (approximately 50 cc of bright red blood) with a decrease in his urinary output. He had been well until six weeks previously when he first noticed night sweats and a constant feeling of tiredness. He also complained of constipation, dark red urine, nauseas and vomiting the day prior to the admission. He denied any smoking or drinking habits. He has a history of exposure to asbestos for 15 years. His physical examination was unremarkable except for mild edema in his lower extremities.

Laboratory analysis:

BLOOD

Creatinine:	6.9	mg/dL
BUN:	74	mg/dL
Bilirubin:	1.4	mg/dL
SGOT:	32	IU/L
SGPT:	40	IU/L
Alkaline phosphatase:	112	IU/L
GGT:	60	IU/L
PT	11	seconds
PTT	25	seconds
Hemoglobin:	8.5	g/dL
Hematocrit:	25	%
MCV:	86	fl
MCH:	29	pg
WBC:	7.2×10^9	u/L
Neutrophils:	61	% PMN
	41	% lymphocytes
Platelets:	2.7×10^9	/Ul
ESR:	75	mm/h

URINE
Urinanalysis: proteinuria+++, hyaline and granular casts +++; RBC +++, WBC ++

CHEST-X-RAY
Flofly infiltrate in both fields, with no cavitation, no masses or pleural effusion. Normal cardiac siluette.

92. Which of the following statements regarding this disease is CORRECT?

a) Increase in gamma globulin and raised alpha-2 globulins is seen in the serum protein electrophoresis
b) A selective humoral deficiency of IgA is present in serum
c) Clonal proliferation of B cell lymphocytes is seen in lymph nodes and bone marrow
d) A neoplastic proliferation of a single clone of plasma cells is responsible of this disease
e) Kidney and lungs present a lineal deposition of anti-basal membrane antibodies

93. The renal failure in this patient:

a) it can be irreversible
b) it is not related to the baseline disease
c) it is caused by the toxic effect of a monoclonal paraprotein
d) it requires a selective measurement of renine and aldosterone levels
e) none of the above

94. If you suspect Wegener's disease, which of the following serum immunologic tests is more sensitive and specific for this diagnosis?

a) ANA
b) Serum ANCA
c) Latex test
d) Antimicrosomal antibodies
e) None of the above

95. The most likely diagnosis is:

a) Dermatomyositis
b) Good pasture syndrome
c) Lupus erythematous systemic
d) Polyarteritis nodosa
e) None of the above

USMLE step 3

CLINICAL SCIENCES

BOOKLET C TEST 3

Questions: 98 Time: 105 minutes

Item 1-2

A 69-year-old white male is brought to the emergency room after having dizziness, palpitations and pressure type chest pain. He has a history of CAD with CABG 10 years ago. He is a heavy smoker and he is taking metoprolol and lasix for hypertension. His physical examination shows: blood pressure 120/70 mm Hg, pulse 170 bpm with normal heart and lungs sounds. An EKG obtained in the emergency room is shown in the figure C.23.

1. The EKG shows:

a) atrial tachycardia
b) atrial fibrillation
c) supraventricular tachycardia
d) ventricular tachycardia
e) ventricular fibrillation

2. The most appropriate therapeutic intervention is:

a) verapamil p.o.
b) adenosine i.v.
c) digoxin i.v.
d) beta-blockers i.v.
e) verapamil i.v.

3. Which of the following statements regarding ulcerative colitis is INCORRECT?

a) Incidence is higher among jews than non-jewish population
b) Involves the caecum and spreads proximally
c) Females are affected more often than males
d) Bimodal age of incidence prevails
e) It is a premalignant disease

4. Which of the following physical signs is LEAST likely to be seen in left heart failure?

a) Crackles throughout lungs
b) Third or fourth heart sound audible
c) Pericardial rub
d) Cardiac enlargement
e) Gallop cadency

5. A 6-year-old boy is admitted for thrombocytopenia, purpura and white blood cell count of 40,000/ul with 90% blast in smear of peripheral blood. He develops intensive headache and he has noted radical changes in his mental status (irritability, coprolalia) with one episode of focal seizure. The most likely diagnostic is:

a) chronic lymphocytic leukemia
b) meningeal carcinomatosis
c) infectious meningitis
d) acute psychosis
e) none of the above

6. Hypercalcemia is most likely to be seen in the following conditions, EXCEPT:

a) sarcoidosis
b) bone metastasis formation
c) hyperparathyroidism
d) carcinoid
e) vitamin D intoxication

7. Which of the following statements regarding hyperosmolar coma in a non-insulin dependent diabetic patient is INCORRECT?

a) It is the result of severe dehydration
b) It may occur in undiagnosed diabetics
c) The resulting osmotic diuresis leads to disproportionate water loss
d) The increase in plasma osmolarity is caused by an increase in the total plasmatic sodium
e) It is rarely seen until the serum glucose level exceeds 800 mg/dl

8. Which of the following interventions in patients with generalized muscle spasm caused by tetanus is INAPPROPRIATE?

a) To administer systemic steroids
b) To clean and to debride the infected site
c) To administer diazepam, muscle relaxants and to isolate the patient
d) To neutralize the tetanus toxin by IM administration of 3,000-10,000 units of human immune globulin
e) To use mechanical ventilation if respiratory muscles are involved

9. Blockade of alpha-adrenergic receptor causes:

a) bronchocontriction
b) reduction in peripheral vascular resistance
c) reflex bradycardia
d) no significant changes
e) none of the above

10. The sedative drug that has the potential risk for addiction is:

a) choral hydrate
b) diphenhydramine
c) glutethimide
d) meprobamate
e) none of the above

Figure C.23

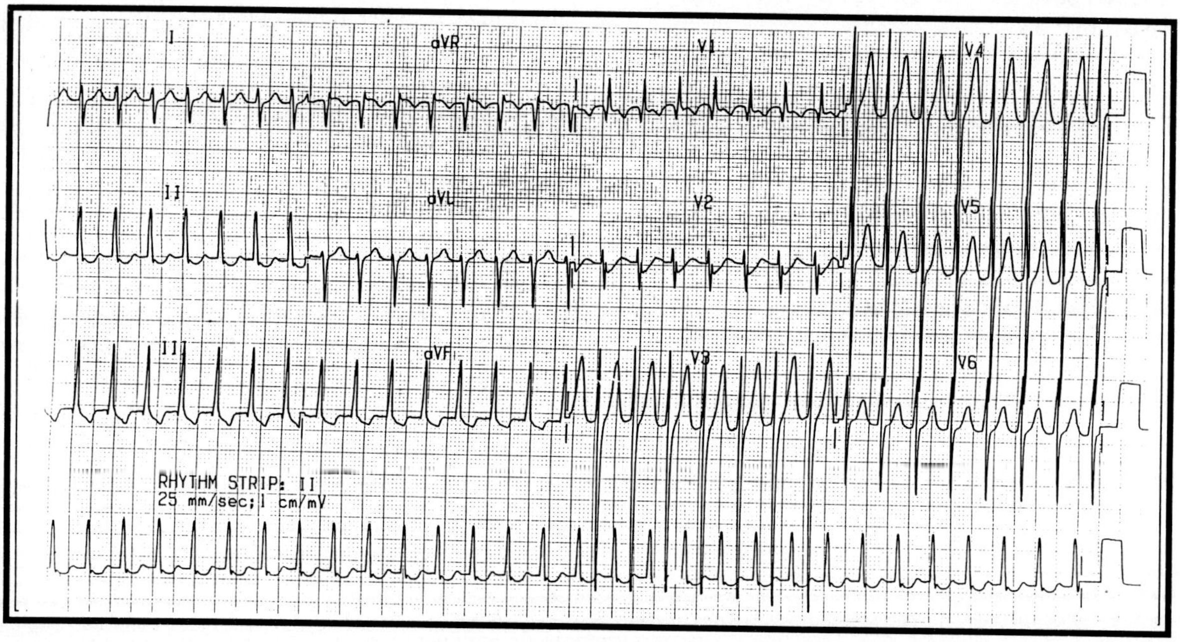

Items 11

The following is an electrocardiogram in a 55-year-old white male who complains of palpitations and dizziness. He has been on quinidine and digital for a previous history of atrial fibrillation. He had a work up for coronary artery disease one year ago showing normal coronary arteries and normal ventricular contractibility. His physical examination is unremarkable except for tachycardia 125 bpm. BP 120/80 mm Hg (see figure C.24).

11. The most likely electrocardiographic diagnostic is:

a) atrial fibrillation
b) atrial flutter
c) idioventricular tachycardia
d) junctional tachycardia
e) frequent premature atrial contractions

Item 12

A 66-year-old while female is seen with fever, nausea and vomiting. Her physical examination reveals mild dehydration, several enlarged lymphadenopathy are palpable with remarkable splenomegaly. A complete blood count shows: WBC 745,000/uL, hemoglobin 10 mg/dL and platelets 68,000/uL. The blood smear is shown in the figure C.25.

12. The most likely diagnosis is:

a) acute myelogenous leukemia
b) acute lymphocytic leukemia
c) hairy cell leukemia
d) chronic lymphocytic leukemia
e) chronic myelocytic leukemia

Item 13-14

A 39-year-old homosexual with HIV infection (CD4 cell count, 250/uL) is admitted to the hospital with a 3-day history of fever (temperature, 103.3°F) and cough with yellow sputum. He was admitted to the hospital six months ago with the same symptoms. His current medications include zidovudine and multivitamins. His physical examination reveals crackles in the left lung. A chest-x-ray and an induced sputum examination are shown in the figures C.26 and C.27 respectively.

13. The most likely cause of this patient's symptoms is:

a) Mycobacterium tuberculosis
b) invasive histoplasmosis
c) Pneumocystis carinii pneumonia
d) pleural effusion caused by Cytomegalovirus
e) pneumonia caused by S. pneumoniae

14. The treatment of choice is:

a) penicillin
b) TMT/SMX
c) itrakonazole
d) amphotericin B
e) erythromycin

Figure C.25

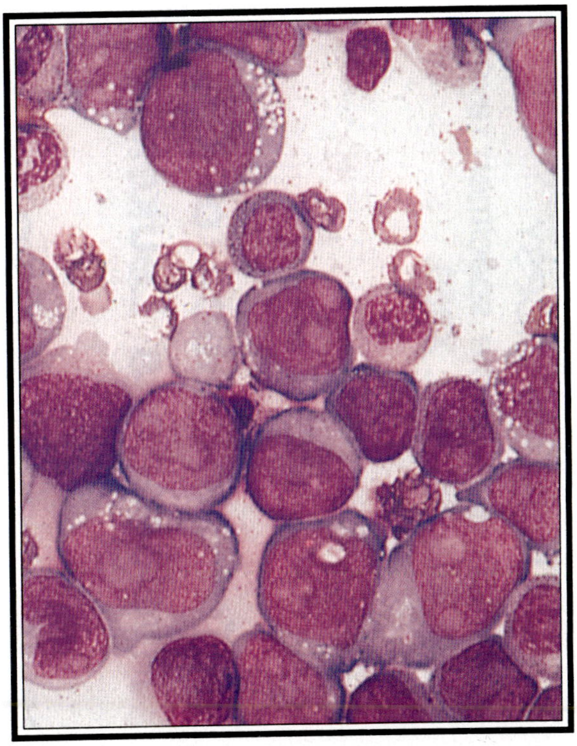

Figure C.24

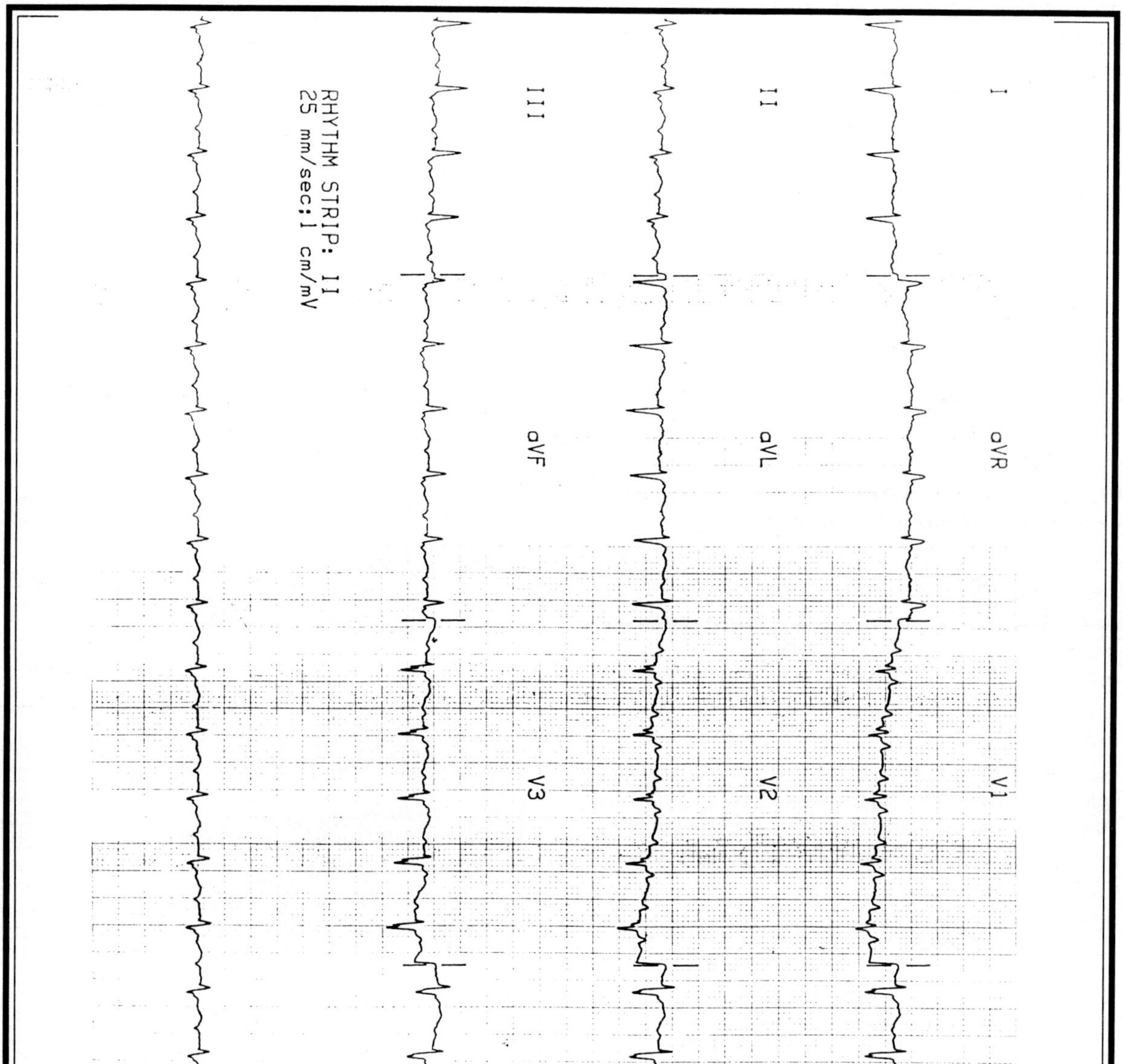
I
II
III
aVR
aVL
aVF
V1
V2
V3
V4
V5
V6
RHYTHM STRIP: II
25 mm/sec;1 cm/mV
.05-40Hz

15. The LEAST common cause of primary amenorrhea is:

a) pelvic inflammatory disease
b) hypothyroidism
c) polycystic ovaric
d) cervical incontinence
e) pituitary hypothalamic dysfunction

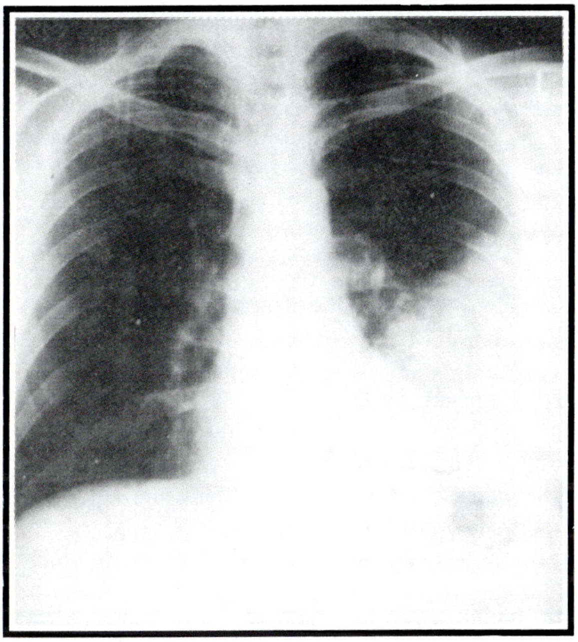

Figure C.26 (top) and C.27 bottom).

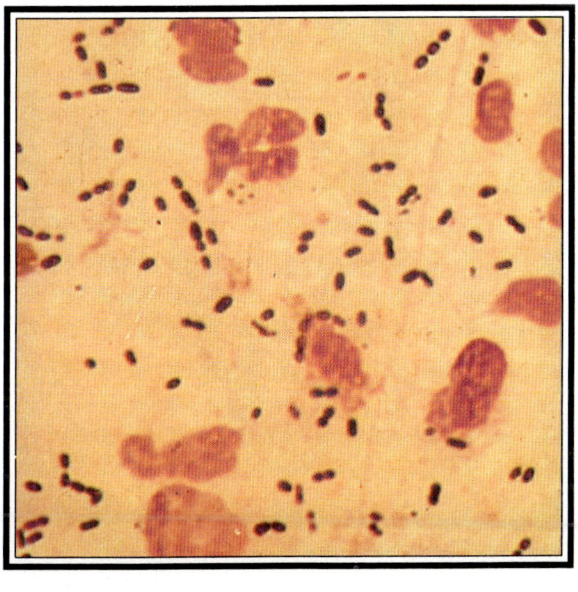

16. Puberty is considered precocious if menarche and secondary sexual characteristics occur before the age of (in years):

a) 7
b) 9
c) 12
d) 14
e) 16

17. Which of the following is the most specific laboratory test in order to differentiate hypercalcemia caused by primary hyperthyroidism from hypercalcemia caused by neoplasia?

a) Low parathohormone level is seen in malignancy
b) Increased levels of alkaline phosphatase is seen in malignancy
c) Normal levels of calcium in urine is seen in primary parathyroidism
d) Prostaglandin inhibitors are effective in treating the hypercalcemia caused by malignancy
e) None of the above

18. Spots of pigmentation around the mouth can be seen in:

a) Crohn's disease
b hereditary hemorrhagic telangiectasia
c) Peutz-Jeghers syndrome
d) psoriasis
e) none of the above

19. The following statements regarding the response to death are correct, EXCEPT:

a) is based on his or her level of awareness
b) children younger than 5 years tend to view death as abandonment
c) middle childhood causes severe anxiety for the loss of loved ones and also fears of mutilation and suffering
d) adolescents fail to appreciate its finality and irreversibility
e) children feel separated

Items 20-23

A 64-year-old white male is seen for pain in the left side of his chest and upper abdomen with general malaise and a skin lesion in the same area (see figure C.28). He denies previous medical diseases or weight loss. His physical examination is unremarkable except for the skin lesion.

20. Which of the following is the most likely diagnosis?

a) Herpes simplex
b) Herpes zoster
c) Rocky mountain fever
d) Impetigo
e) Mycosis fungoide

21. Which of the following is an UNCOMMON complication of this clinical picture?

a) Postherpetic neuralgia
b) Pneumonitis
c) Meningoencephalitis
d) Leukemia
e) Hepatitis

22. Which of the following statements regarding this disease is INCORRECT?

a) Pain may precede the development of lesions by 48-72 hours
b) Acute neuritis and postherpetic neuralgia are more common in children
c) In immunocompromised patients the syndrome is more severe
d) Cutaneous dissemination occurs in about 40% of immunocompromised patients
e) Disseminated infection is rarely fatal

23. Prophylaxis for susceptible patients with significant exposure is based on:

a) acyclovir i.v.
b) vidarabine i.v.
c) varicella-zoster immune globulin
d) amitriptyline hydrochloride p.o.
e) steroids p.o.

24. The following statements regarding the diffusion capacity of the lungs are correct, EXCEPT:

a) It is measured using carbon monoxide (CO)
b) It is increased during exercise due to a recruitment of capillaries
c) It is increased in emphysema
d) It is reduced in restrictive lung disease
e) It can be normal or increased in alveolar pulmonary hemorrhage

25. Residual volume is most probable increased in patients with:

a) emphysema
b) restrictive lung disease
c) pneumonia
d) asbestosis
e) pulmonary fibrosis

26. Fluid volume of the pleural cavity may increase due to:

a) lymphatic obstruction
b) decrease in pleural blood flow
c) decrease in pleural capillary pressure
d) increase in capillary oncotic pressure
e) none of the above

Figure C.28

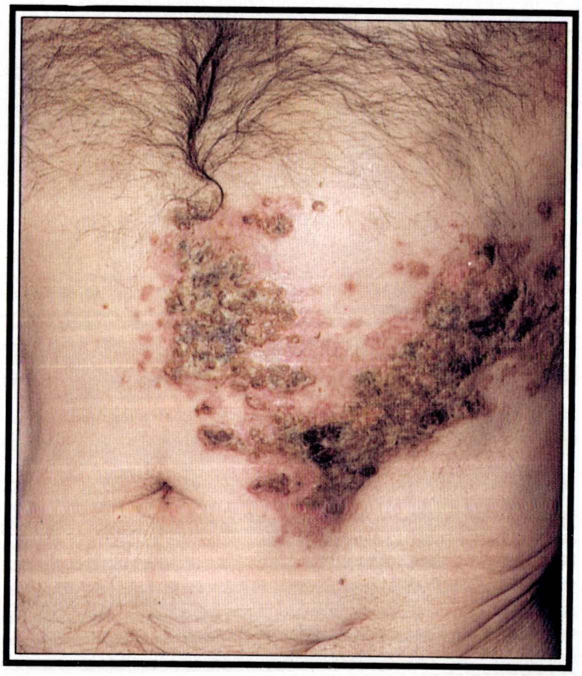

27. The following statements regarding the autonomic nervous system are correct, EXCEPT:

a) blood vessel sympathetic stimulation causes 50% of the maximal vasoconstrictor activity in most of the vascular beds
b) after sympathetic denervation, receptors develop over the entire membrane causing the end of organs to be extremely sensitive to any circulating catecholamines
c) alpha-receptors are stimulated most strongly by epinephrine and norepinephrine causing vasoconstriction
d) beta-2 receptors are located in myocardium and stimulation causes negative inotropic and chronotropic responses

Items 28-30

Match the following ear disorders with their clinical presentations.

a) External otitis
b) Cerumen impaction
c) Acute otitis media
d) Serous otitis media
e) None of the above

28. «Blocked» painless ear with canal clear and dull immobile tympanic membrane.

29. Painful ear with strong evidence of inflamed tympanic membrane.

30. Pain or itching of the ear canal with inflamed canal and normal tympanic membrane.

31. Meconium aspiration syndrome is MOST likely to be associated with the following, EXCEPT:

a) placental insufficiency
b) cord disorders
c) hypertension
d) preterm pregnancy
e) fetal anoxia

32. Hydramnios is LEAST frequently associated with:

a) esophageal atresia
b) spina bifida
c) pulmonary hypoplasia
d) renal hyperplasia
e) anencephalous

33. Which of the following interventions is LEAST likely to correct the luteal phase defect in an infertile female?

a) Clomiphene citrate
b) Hormone chorionic gonadotrophic
c) Postovulatory progesterone supplementation
d) Bromocryptine

34. Surgical patients with anergy:

a) they should receive stimulants of the immune system
b) they should receive preoperative hyperalimentation
c) they should receive preoperative anti-pseudomona antibiotics
d) they are less susceptible to infectious complications in the postoperative period
e) none of the above

35. Genuine stress incontinence:

a) is also referred to as unstable bladder
b) is secondary to inflammation, tumors, or lack of estrogen
c) is the most common cause of incontinence
d) patients have a sudden inability to control their bladder followed by a delayed loss of urine
e) none of the above

36. Incontinence caused by detrusor dyssynergia:

a) can be caused by uninhibited bladder contractions
b) the patient has a sudden inability to control the bladder followed by a delayed loss of urine
c) a strong sensory input from the bladder secondary to inflammation, tumors, or lack of estrogen may cause the urge incontinence
d) may occur following pelvic surgery
e) All of the above

37. The causes of false positives oral cholecystography are the following, EXCEPT:

a) Serum bilirubin greater than 1.8 mg/dL
b) Emesis or intestinal malabsorption of the dye
c) Inadequate hepatic excretion
d) Malnutrition
e) Failure of the patient to take the pills

Items 38

A 60-year-old white female asymptomatic is seen in the clinic for a routine check up. She has a history of hypertension and she was admitted to the hospital four years ago, after having heart problems. An EKG was obtained (see figure C.29).

38. What is the MOST likely diagnosis?

a) an old anterior myocardial infarct
b) an acute Q-wave inferior myocardial infarct
c) a subendocardial myocardial infarct
d) a posterior myocardial infarct
e) an old inferior myocardial infarct

Item 39-41

A 29-year-old black male complains of palpitations several times during the day with occasional dyspnea during exercise. An EKG was obtained (see figure C.30). His physical examination shows tachycardia (160 bpm), BP 140/85 mm Hg with normal lung and heart sounds.

39. The EKG is compatible with:

a) preexcitation syndrome
b) thyrotoxicosis
c) essential hypertension
d) sinus tachycardia
e) none of the above

40. The most appropriate treatment may include:

a) intravenous digital
b) procainamide
c) intravenous labetalol
d) intravenous verapamil
e) immediate direct-current cardioversion

41. The following statements regarding this patient's disease are correct, EXCEPT :

a) aortic regurgitation
b) pulmonary regurgitation
c) mitral stenosis
d) hypertrophic cardiomyopathy
e) dilated cardiomyopathy

Item 42

A 41-year-old white male presents painful swelling and redness in the right knee and both ankles. The following day he noted several small lesions in both lower extremities (see figure C.31). He also complains of several days of nausea, vomiting and one episode of coffee ground emesis. He has no previous medical history. He denies alcohol or drug abuse. His physical examination is unremarkable except for evidences of arthritis in the knees and the skin lesions shown in the figure C.31. The most likely diagnosis is:

a) Henoch-Schonlein purpura
b) chronic urticaria
c) dermatomyositis
d) rheumatic polymyalgia
e) none of the above

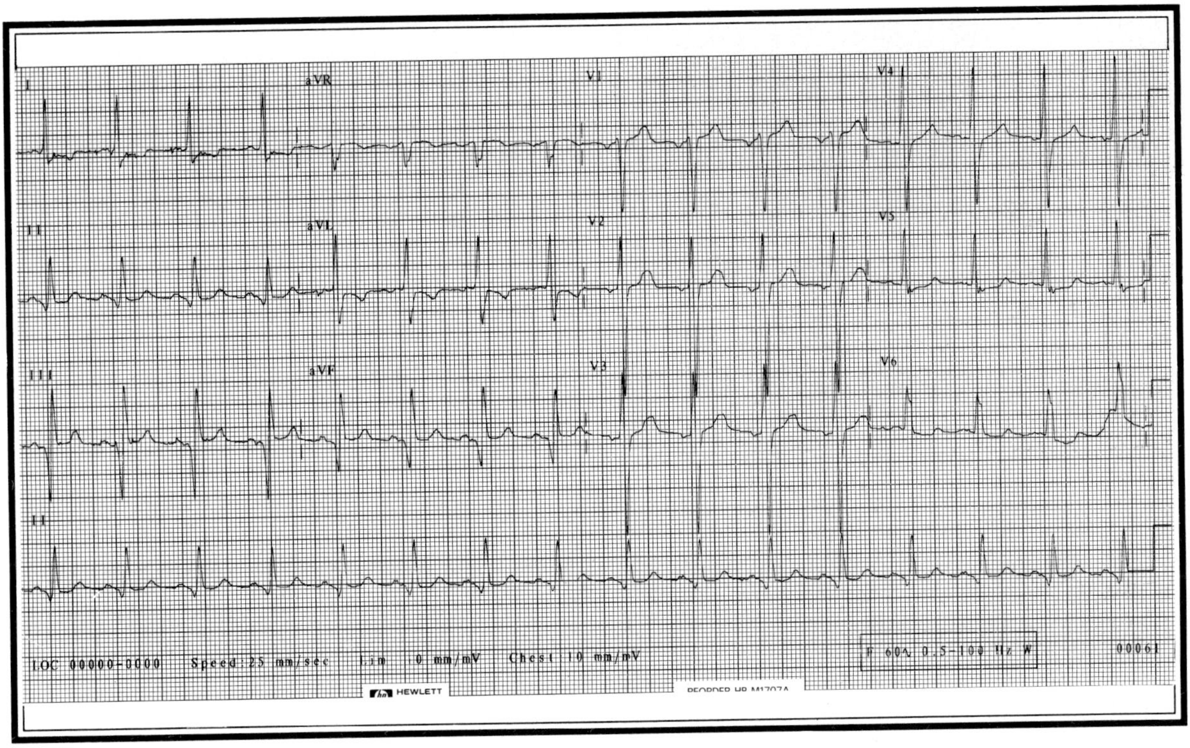

FIgure C.29

FIgure C.30

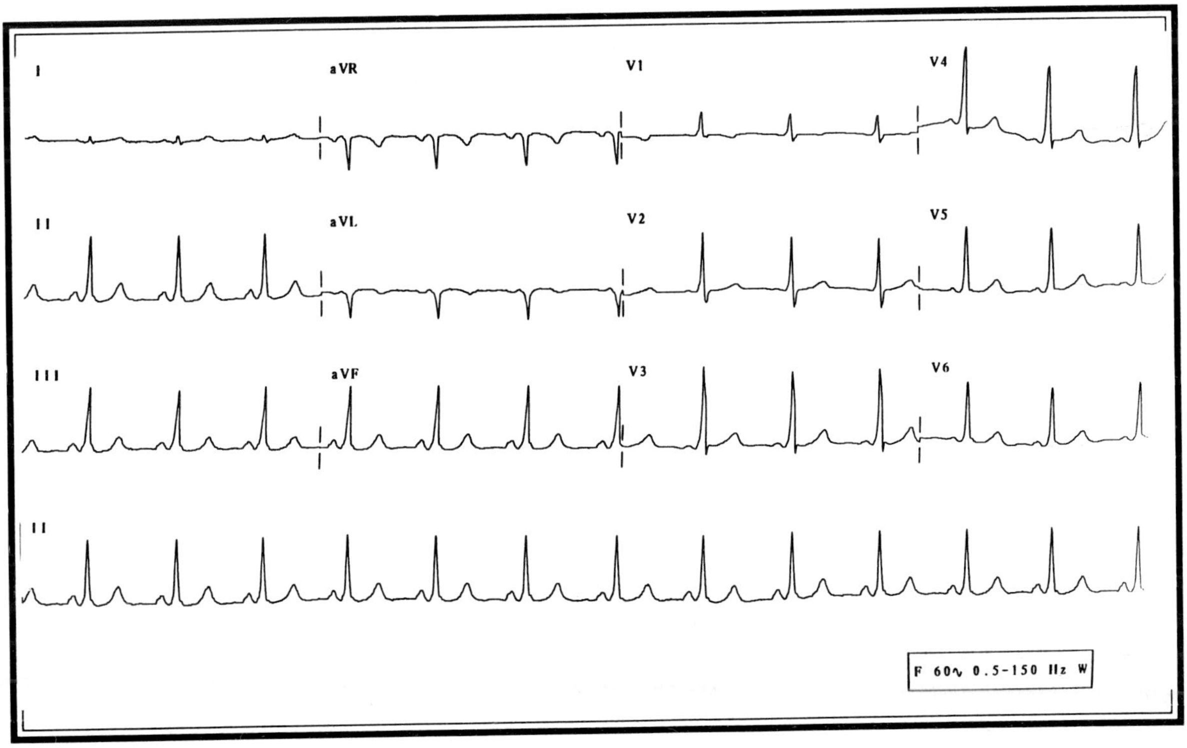

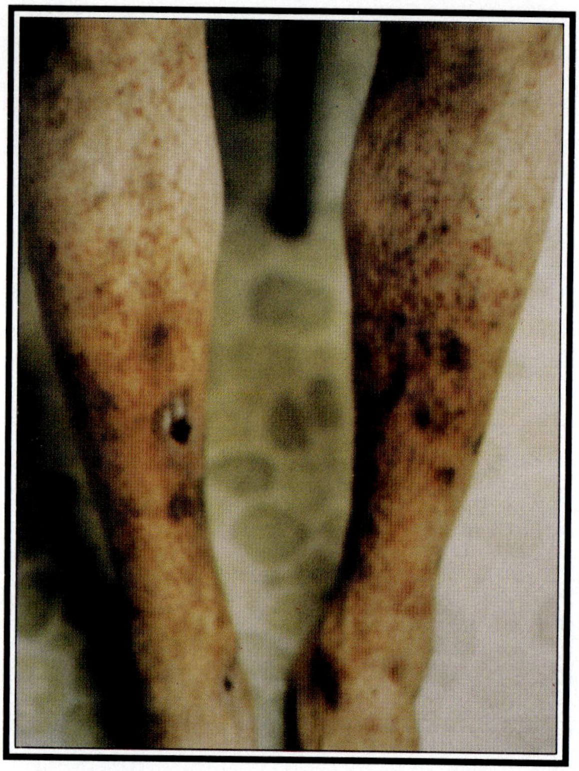

Figure C.31

Items 43-44

A 72-year-old white male with a history of hypertension, diabetes mellitus and CAD, status post CABG six years ago, complains of palpitations, shortness of breath, cough and wheezing. He also noticed orthopnea and paroxysmal nocturnal dyspnea worsening during the last week. He is cyanotic, BP was 150/70 mm Hg and pulse was 138 bpm irregular. Jugulars were engorged and bilateral fine crackles with inspiratory wheezes were auscultated in both lungs. S3 heart sound was present with bilateral pedal edema. A previous echocardiogran showed dilated chambers with 30% ejection fraction. A chest-x-ray was obtained (see figure C.32).

43. The clinical picture is compatible with:

a) pulmonary emboli
b) biventricular congestive heart failure
c) right ventricular failure
d) ventricular aneurysm
e) lower respiratory infection

44. The following should be included in the treatment of this patient, EXCEPT:

a) ACE-inhibitors
b) digitalis and diuretics
c) anticoagulation
d) aspirin
e) verapamil

Items 45-50

Match the electrolyte disorder with its most common clinical presentation.

a) Hyponatremia
b) Hypercalcemia
c) Hypomagnesemia
d) Hypernatremia
e) Hyperkalemia

Figure C.32

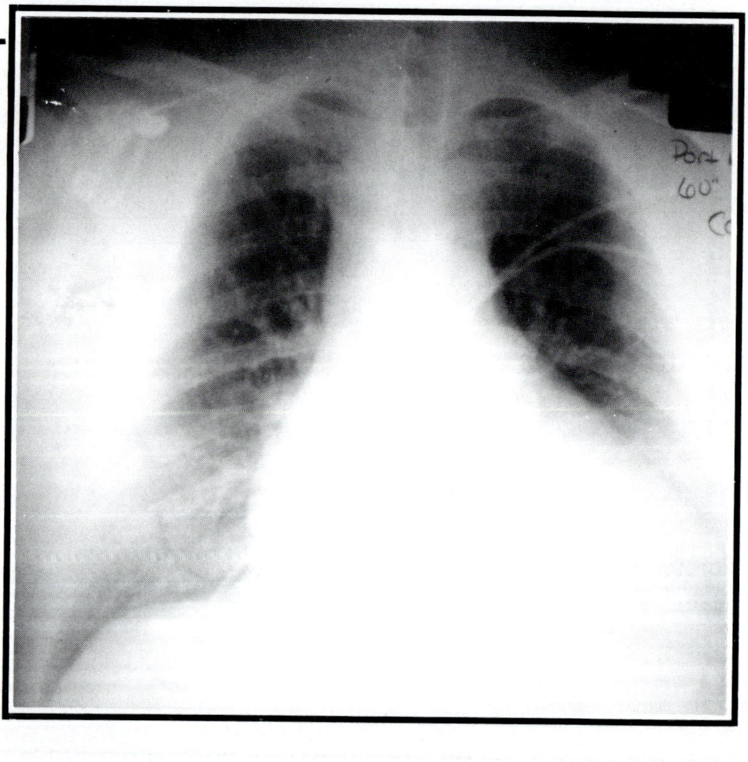

45. It is most commonly seen with severe dehydration.

46. It is most commonly seen in syndrome of inappropriate antidiuretic hormone secretion (SIADH).

47. It usually occurs with malignancy and metastatic spreading and in presence of an excess in parathohormone.

48. It is a frequent electrolyte abnormality seen in alcoholic intoxication and in patients treated with chemotherapy.

49. It is seen in patients treated with spironolactone.

50. It should be suspected in patients with anorexia, nausea, thirst, polyuria, polydipsia, headaches, constipation, mood changes and shortened QT interval in the EKG.

Items 51-53

A 62 year-old white female is admitted for rapid growth of a mass in her neck. She experiences increasing fatigue, cold intolerance, alopecia and shortness of breath. In the clinic she presents stridor.

Laboratory:

Free thyroxine index	0.6	(low)
Thyroid stimulating hormone (TSH)	60 uU	(high)
(normal serum TSH< 3 uU)		
Thyroidal microsomal antibodies	positive	

A needle-aspirated specimen from thyroid tissue is shown in the figure C.33.

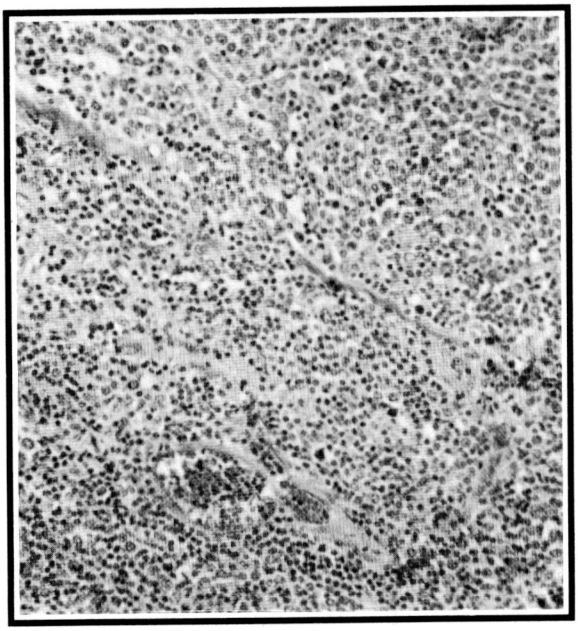

Figure C.33

51. Laboratory analysis is compatible with:

a) primary hypothyroidism
b) Hashimoto's thyroiditis
c) Graves' disease
d) medular carcinoma of the thyroids
e) none of the above

52. To confirm the mechanical obstruction caused by the mass, which of the following tests is most appropriate?

a) ABG's
b) A pulmonary flow-volume loop study
c) DLCO
d) Spirometry with and without bronchodilators
e) Lateral chest x-ray

53. Which of the following statements regarding this clinical picture is INCORRECT?

a) CT scan is useful in evaluating the obstruction and size of the infiltrating mass
b) Iodine uptake scans shows low radioactive uptake (5% in 24 hrs)
c) Treatment should include replacement with levothyroxine hormone
d) Medular carcinoma of the thyroids is most likely to develop in the course of Hashimoto's thyroiditis
e) Surgical partial thyroidectomy and release of the obstruction is indicated

54. Which of the following is NOT a common side effect of anti-cholinergic drugs?

a) Dry mouth
b) Blurring of vision
c) Bradycardia
d) Constipation
e) Restlessness, confusion, and delirium

55. Which of the following is an extrinsic factor that triggers the coagulation cascade?

a) Platelet factor 3
b) Fibrin
c) Thromboplastin
d) Factor XII
e) Factor V

56. Which of the following is a potential complication of the percutaneous transluminal coronary angioplasty (PTCA)?

a) Coronary artery dissection
b) Occlusion of coronary arteries
c) Spasm of coronary arteries
d) Myocardial infarct during the procedure
e) Dressler's syndrome

57. Which of the following statements regarding the radionuclide diagnosis of myocardial infarct is INCORRECT?

a) Technetium-99-labeled pyrophosphate is positive between 2-5 days following the myocardial infarct
b) Exercise thallium-201 is useful in the evaluation of angina pectoris
c) Technetium-99m-pyrophosphate-labeled red blood cells (MUGA) is useful in assessing the right and left ventricular ejection fraction
d) MUGA is also indicted in assessing the cardiac size and ventricular ejection fraction of patients in atrial fibrillation
e) "Cold spots" in the myocardial perfusion with Thallium 201 are seen in areas of old infarction

58. In genuine stress incontinence (GSI), the loss of urine:

a) occurs after performing a physical activity
b) may be caused by coughing or sneezing
c) may be associated to pelvic relaxation problems (cystocele, rectocele)
d) follows physical activity or occurs while at rest
e) may be associated with intercourse

Items 59-61

A 54-year-old white male is seen for the skin lesions shown in the figure C.34. He denied any previous medical diseases or weight loss. He said that he has had those lesions for years and usually the skin looks worse when he is exposed to sunlight or when he drinks alcohol. His physical examination is unremarkable except for blistering skin lesions with hyperpigmentation and ulceration, present in face, forehead and forearms.

59. Which of the following is the most likely diagnosis?

a) Polymorphous light eruption
b) Scleroderma
c) Tuberous sclerosis
d) Intermittent acute porphyria
e) Porphyria Cutanea Tarda

60. Which of the following is NOT a common feature of this disease?

a) Deficiency of uroporphyrinogen decarboxylase
b) Neurologic and psychiatric disturbances
c) Photosensitivity
d) Increased fragility of skin
e) Liver disease

61. The management of this patient may include the following, EXCEPT:

a) abstinence from alcohol
b) avoid sunlight
c) phlebotomy
d) topical steroids
e) chloroquine

62. Primary carcinoma of the esophagus:

a) squamous cell type usually occurs in the lower esophagus
b) adenocarcinomas occurs usually in the upper esophagus
c) it may be associated with smoking and alcohol abuse
d) they are «good prognosis tumors
e) they do not grow into the mediastinum

63. Which of the following symptoms and signs is NOT characteristic of gastroesophageal reflux with esophagitis?

a) Substernal burning discomfort after meals
b) Regurgitation of gastric juice at night
c) Dysphagia
d) Pain is relieved by sitting up
e) Recurrent episodes of cough

64. Which of the following is NOT an alcohol-induced organic mental disorder?

a) Alcohol intoxication
b) Elective mutism
c) Korsakoff's syndrome
d) Delirium tremens
e) Withdrawal delirium

65. Which of the following is(are) a pathogenic mechanism(s) of community acquired pneumonias?

a) Aspiration
b) Hematogenous spreading
c) Inhalation of an infectious aerosol
d) All of the above

Item 66-67

A 72-year-old white male with a history of hypertension, diabetes mellitus and coronary artery disease (CAD), status post CABG six years ago, complains of palpitations and shortness of breath getting worse in the last three days. His BP 160/100 mm Hg, pulse 138 bpm irregular. Jugulars are engorged and bilateral fine crackles are auscultated in both lungs. S3 heart sound and bilateral pedal edema are present. An EKG was obtained (see figure C.35).

66. The EKG shows:

a) atrial fibrillation
b) ventricular tachycardia
c) idioventricular tachycardia
d) junctional tachycardia
e) supraventricular tachycardia

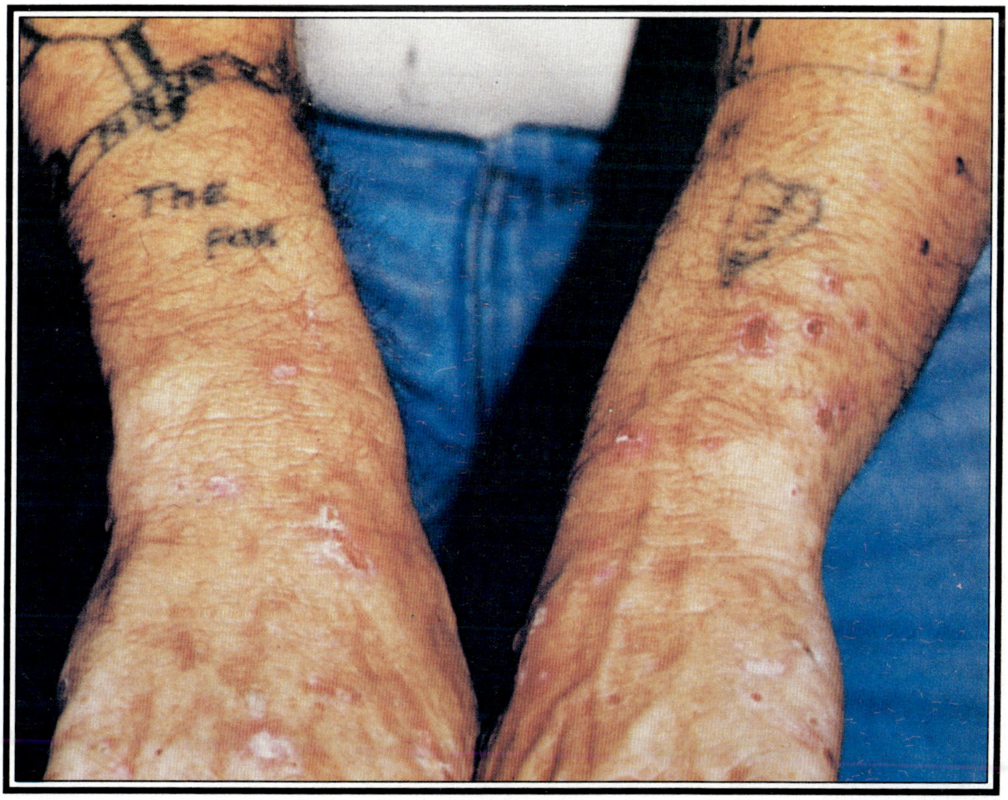

Figure C.34

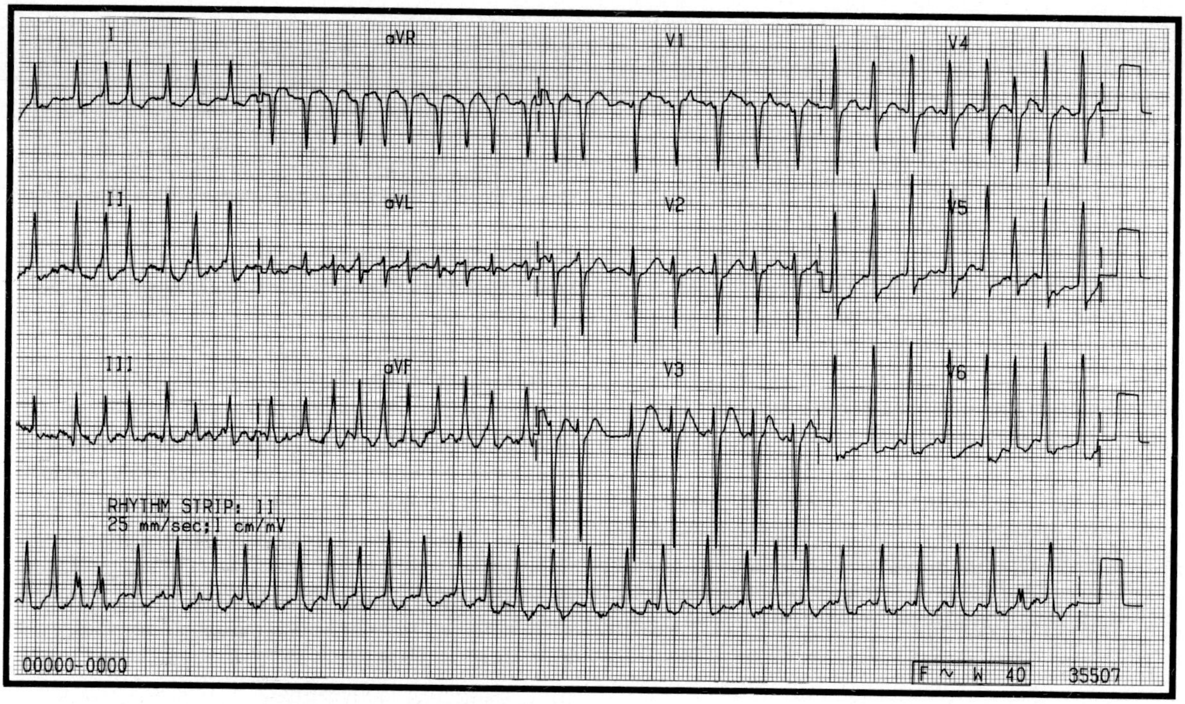

FIgure C.35

FIgure C.36

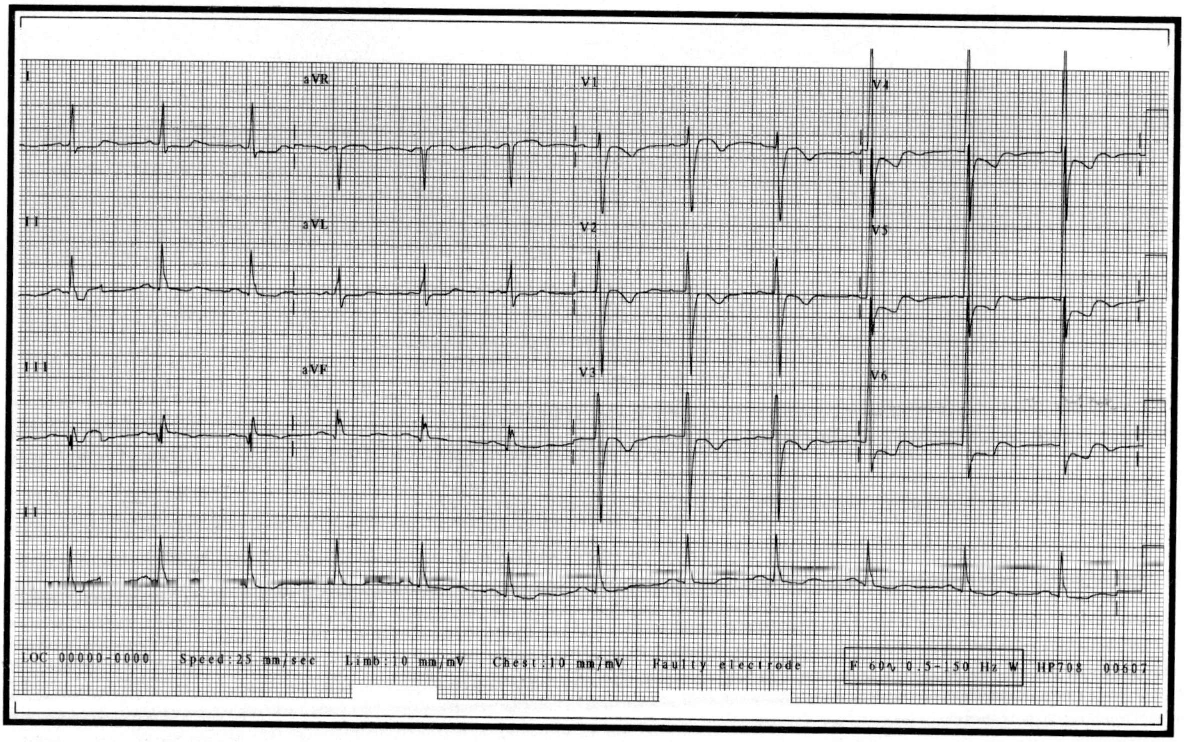

67. The most appropriate therapeutic intervention is:

a) heart catheterization
b) digitalis and diuretics
c) to start with procainamide
d) to start an infusion of amiodarone
e) to start quinidine

Items 68-70

Match the features of the following abdominal clinical findings with their disease.

a) Mesenteric vascular occlusion
b) Paralytic ileus
c) Large bowel obstruction
d) Appendicitis
e) None of the above

68. Absence of bowel sounds in patient after a recent operation with prolonged return of bowel function. KUB shows both small and large bowel gas without differential air/fluid levels.

69. An elderly patient with recent myocardial infarct presents sudden, severe abdominal pain an abdominal tenderness out of proportion to physical findings. Laboratory tests: markedly elevated WBC count, hyperamylasemia, unexplained, persistent metabolic acidosis.

70. Patient of 60-year-old with marked abdominal distention before significant symptoms appear. KUB shows distended gas-filled colon.

71. The recommended treatment to prevent diverticulitis in a patient with multiple diverticula in the colon is:

a) a diet high in fiber
b) prophylaxis with antibiotics
c) low doses of NSAIDs
d) steroids per oral
e) metamucil

72. The following are indications for surgery in Crohn's disease, EXCEPT:

a) enteroenteral fistulas
b) abscess
c) intestinal obstruction
d) cecal involvement
e) ileocolic fistulas

Item 73-75

A 69-year-old white female is brought to the emergency room with chest pain and shortness of breath. She complains of progressive chest pain, pressure type radiated to her left arm specially when she walks during the last 5 days. The pain is usually released after one or two nitroglycerin sublingual. Last night the pain become constant in the middle of the chest. She has a history of an inferior myocardial infarct one year ago and non-insulin dependent diabetes mellitus. She is taking aspirin, metoprolol, diabeta and long acting nitrites.The physical examination shows a patient resting comfortable, BP 100/60 mm Hg, pulse 75 bpm regular, afebrile, with normal heart sounds and few bibasal fine crackles in both lungs. The EKG is shown in the figure C.36.

Laboratory analysis:

BLOOD		
Sodium	138	mEq/L
Potassium	4.0	mEq/L
Glucose	190	mg/dL
CPK	430	U/L
CPK-MB	54	U/L
LDH	200	U/L
SGOT	80	U/L
SGPT	56	U/L
WBC	9,400	cells/uL
Hemoglobin	13	mg/dL
Platelets	260,000	platelets/uL

73. Patient is having:

a) an acute anterior myocardial infarct
b) an acute Q-wave anterior myocardial infarct
c) a subendocardial myocardial infarct
d) a posterior myocardial infarct
e) an inferior myocardial infarct

74. Appropriate interventions should include the following, EXCEPT

a) calcium channel blocker agents
b) aspirin
c) heparin
d) thrombolytic therapy
e) morphine

75. In this patient:

a) early thrombolytic therapy can reduce infarct size
b) diltiazem given within 72 hours may prevent later reinfarction and recurrent angina
c) thrombolysis should be given immediately
d) beta-adrenergic blockers reduce myocardial oxygen consumption but increase the mortality rate
e) subsequent infarction or coronary events are unlikely in this patient

76. Typical clinical findings suspicious of pheochromocytoma are the following, EXCEPT:

a) labile severe hypertension
b) paroxysmal hypertension
c) headaches
d) nephrotic syndrome
e) abnormal glucose tolerance

77. The following findings suggest Cushing's syndrome, EXCEPT:

a) galactorrhea
b) truncal obesity
c) striae in the skin
d) weakness and muscle wasting
e) abnormal menses

78. Clubbing and bibasilar crackles in the auscultation of the chest is most likely seen in:

a) acute bronchitis
b) interstitial lung disease
c) endobronchial tumors
d) pulmonary tuberculosis
e) none of the above

79. Surgical drainage is clearly indicated in all the following conditions, EXCEPT:

a) subphrenic abscess
b) bacterial peritonitis
c) purulent pericarditis
d) fibroexudative pulmonary tuberculosis
e) septic arthritis

Item 80- 81

A 64-year-old black male complains of dizziness, palpitations and chest pain during the last 5 hours before arriving to the emergency room. He denies any shortness of breath, orthopnea or paroxysmal nocturnal dyspnea. His physical examination is unremarkable, blood pressure 90/50 mm Hg, pulse 170 bpm. His past medical history is significant for two episodes of myocardial infarcts, hypertension, diabetes mellitus and hypercholesterolemia. He is on lasix, digoxin and capoten. His physical examination is remarkable for tachycardia, tachypnea with cold and clammy extremities. An EKG obtained in the emergency room is shown in the figure C.37.

80. The EKG shows:

a) atrial tachycardia
b) atrial fibrillation
c) supraventricular tachycardia
d) ventricular tachycardia
e) ventricular fibrillation

81. The most appropriate therapeutic intervention is:

a) verapamil p.o.
b) D.C. cardioversion
c) digoxin i.v.
d) beta-blockers i.v.
e) adenosine i.v.

82. Necrotizing fascitis is caused by the following microorganisms, EXCEPT:

a) Microaerophilic streptococci
b) Staphylococci sp.
c) gram negative bacilli
d) all aerobic streptococcus
e) clostridial microorganism

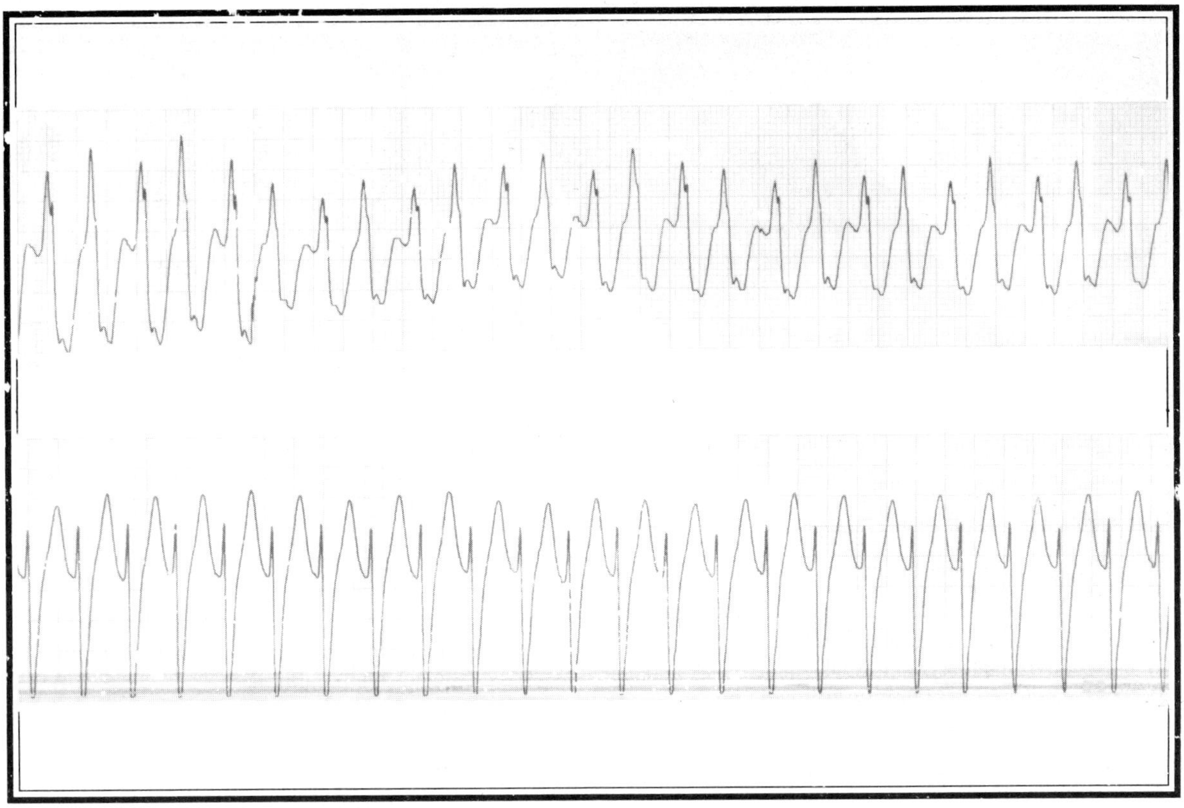

Figure C.37

Item 83-85

A 49-year-old white male previously in good health, is admitted to the hospital after having several episodes of cough with hemoptysis. He denied any TB contact and he lost 15 pounds in the last 3 months. He is a heavy smoker and he has worked as a car salesman for 20 years. His physical examination is unremarkable except for an emphysematous lung with decrease in alveolar lung sounds. A chest-x-ray and CT scan are obtained (see figures C.38 and C.39).

Laboratory analysis:

BLOOD

Sodium	128	mEq/L
Potassium	3.5	mEq/L
Chloride	99	mEq/L
Calcium	11.2	mg /L
Magnesium	1.4	mg/dL
Bicarbonate	22	mEq/L
Albumin	2.9	g/dl
Total Protein	6.1	g/dl
WBC	7,400	cells/uL
Hemoglobin	12	mg/dL

ABG's (room air)

pH	7.38	
pO2	68	mm Hg
pCO2	41	mm Hg

83. The most likely diagnosis is:

a) right lower lobe pneumonia
b) lung carcinoma
c) diaphragmatic hernia
d) lung abscess
e) right pleural effusion

84. The next diagnostic intervention is:

a) to obtain a bronchoscopy and biopsies
b) thoracotomy and biopsies
c) mediastinoscopy
d) fine needle aspiration
e) calcitonine i.v.

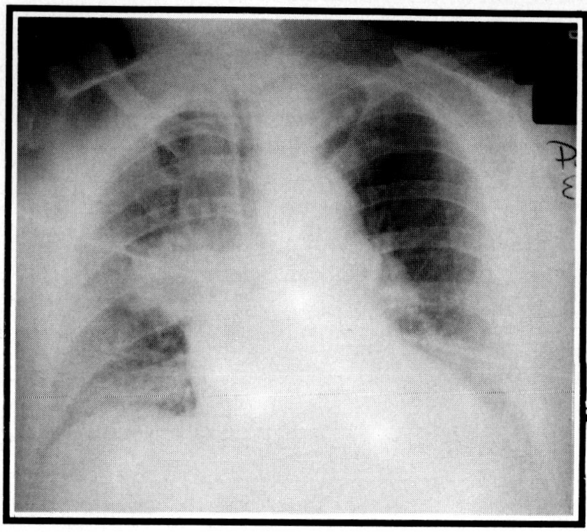

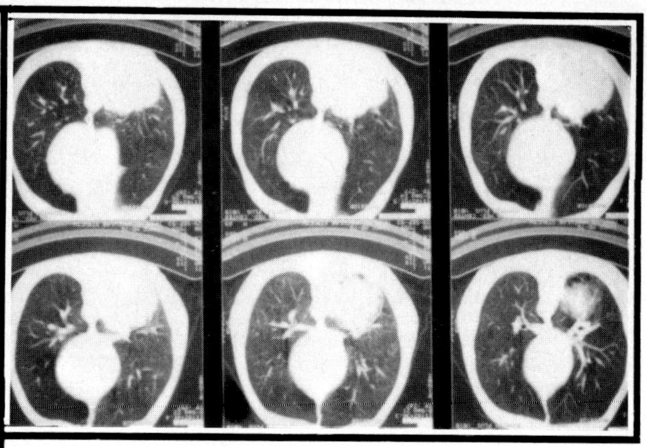

Figures C.38 (left) and C.39 (right).

85. In order to correct the hypercalcemia:

a) a trial of i.v. steroids should be started
b) parathyroidectomy is required
c) an adequate i.v. hydration followed by furosemide should be started
d) a radiation therapy of the lungs should be started immediately
e) none of the above

86. Most likely this patient's hypercalcemia represents:

a) a complication of the bacterial infection
b) a complication of the parasitic infection
c) a manifestation of an epidermoid carcinoma
d) a manifestation of an adenocarcinoma
e) a laboratory error

87. Which of the following statements regarding infective endocarditis is INCORRECT?

a) It usually occurs in an underlying valvular disease
b) The endothelium on the damaged valve leads to the formation of the vegetation
c) The vegetations develop at sites where a regurgitant jet of blood strikes
d) It is an unusual cause of glomerulonephritis
e) The vast majority of patients with tricuspid endocarditis develop pneumonia

88. The most common congenital heart defect with permanent right to left shunt is:

a) patent ductus arteriosus
b) atrial septal defect
c) tetralogy of Fallot
d) ventricular septal defect
e) aortic stenosis

89. Small bowel obstruction may present:

a) Murphy's sign
b) high-pitched, «tinkling» bowel sounds
c) absence of abdominal sounds
d) palpable mass in abdomen
e) none of the above

90. Emphysema can be associated or caused by the following, EXCEPT:

a) air pollution
b) cigarette smoking
c) oxidants that block the antiprotease activity in alveolar spaces
d) increase in the alveolar surface available for gas exchange
e) alpha1-antitrypsin deficiency

91. Naloxone:

a) can cause respiratory depression in normal individuals
b) usually induces tolerance and physical dependence
c) is used to reverse the coma and respiratory intoxication of heroin overdose
d) has a long latency (12-24 hrs) after intravenous administration
e) none of the above

92. Pulmonary edema can be seen under the following conditions, EXCEPT:

a) congestive heart failure
b) volume overload
c) mitral stenosis
d) decrease in capillary hydrostatic pressure
e) acute myocardial infarct

93. Pneumonia caused by Mycoplasma pneumonie:

a) presents non-caseating granuloma formation in the lung
b) can present red cell clumping under microscopic examination of blood smears
c) may present hypercalcemia
d) a normal or low titer in serum of cold agglutinins is usually present
e) none of the above

94. The following conditions may cause or precipitate ischemic heart disease, EXCEPT:

a) thromboembolic event
b) coronary artery spasm
c) coronary arteritis
d) hypothyroidism
e) atherosclerotic heart disease

Item 95-97

A 61-year-old white male previously in good health, is admitted to the hospital after having several episodes of cough with hemoptysis, progressive shortness of breath and swelling in both legs. He denied any TB contacts or loss of weight. He is a heavy smoker and he works as a teacher. His physical examination shows cyanosis, BP 100/60 mm Hg, respiration rate 32/minute, jugulars engorged and trachea in normal position. His left lung does not expand in inspiration with dullness and no sounds are auscultable, except for egophony in the upper left chest. Right lung sounds are normal. Heart sounds are distant and significant edema in the lower extremities is seen. A chest-x-ray and CT scan are obtained (see figures C.40 and C.41).

Laboratory analysis:

BLOOD		
Sodium	128	mEq/L
Potassium	3.5	mEq/L
Chloride	99	mEq/L
Calcium	8.9	mg /dL
Magnesium	1.2	mg/dL
Bicarbonate	18	mEq/L
Albumin	2.9	g/dL
Total Protein	5.1	g/dL
WBC	9,300	cells/uL
Hemoglobin	11	mg/dL

ABG's (room air)		
pH	7.42	
pO2	59	mm Hg
pCO2	29	mm Hg

95. The most likely diagnosis is:

a) left side pneumonia
b) left lung empyema
c) left diaphragmatic hernia
d) left lung collapse
e) left side pleural effusion and atelectasis

96. The next diagnostic intervention is:

a) to obtain a bronchoscopy plus biopsies of the lesions
b) thoracotomy and biopsies
c) thoracocentesis with fluid analysis
d) fine needle aspiration
e) blood cultures

97. You may suspect:

a) congestive heart failure
b) cardiac tamponade
c) airway obstruction
d) diaphragm perforation
e) mediastinitis

98. Which of the following statements regarding the inflammatory bowel disease is INCORRECT?

a) Rectal bleeding is unusual in Crohn's disease but common in chronic ulcerative colitis
b) The findings of abdominal mass and anal complications (fissure, fistula) are more common in Crohn's disease
c) Terminal ileal involvement, skip areas, internal fistulas, and thumb printing are all rare or absent in chronic ulcerative colitis but common in Crohn's disease.
d) Granulomas in the intestinal wall and adjacent lymph nodes are absent in ulcerative colitis but occur in 60% of patients with Crohn s disease
e) The colonic appearance of Crohn's disease is that of focal, predominantly right-sided disease. The mucosa is cobblestone in appearance with transverse ulcerations in affected areas

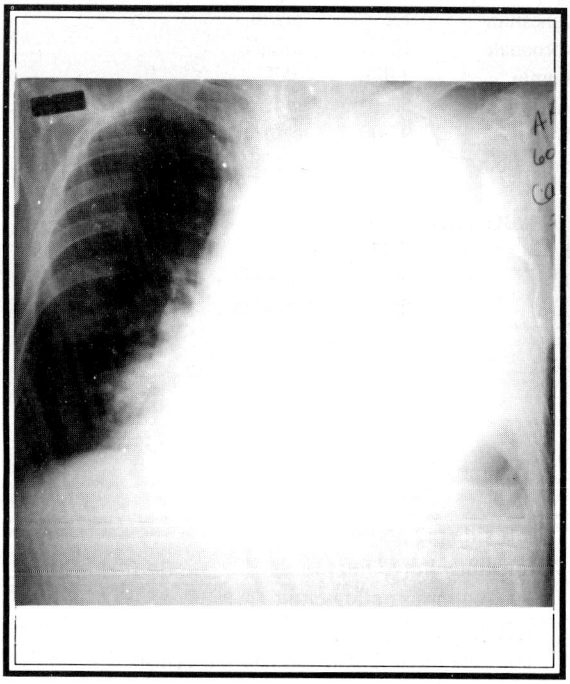

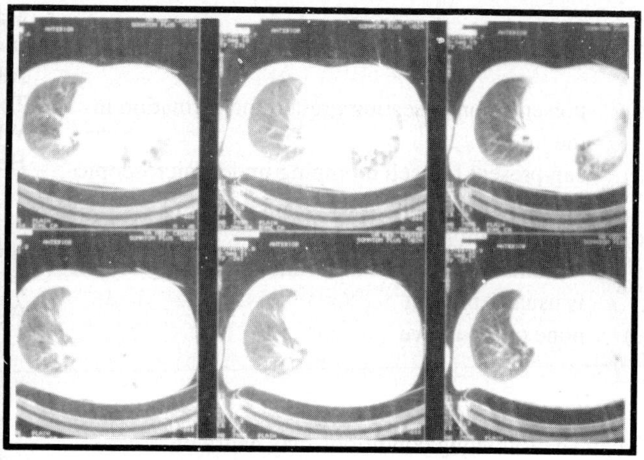

Figures C.40 and C.41

USMLE step 3

ANSWERS

BOOKLET C TEST 1

1. E; 2.A; 3.C; 4.D

Causes of impotence

Organic causes of impotence
- Anterior temporal lobe lesions
- Spinal cord lesions
- Autonomic neuropathy

Vascular disorders (Leriche's syndrome, pelvic vascular insufficiency)
Sickle cell anemia
Endocrine (diabetes mellitus, hypogonadism, hyper-prolactinemia, adrenal insufficiency, feminizing tumors, hypo-hyperthyroidism)
Urogenital (trauma, castration, priapism)
Systemic illness
Drugs (alcohol, barbiturates, spironolactones, anticholinergics, estrogens, guanethidine, reserpine, methyldopa, ketoconazole, phenothiazines, butyrophenones, thiothixenes, tricyclic antidepressants, monoamine oxidase inhibitors, heroin, methadone, morphine, cocaine, amphetamines)
Psychogenic

Psychogenic is one of the mayor causes of impotence. Fear, depression, anger, guilt, anxiety and problems with interpersonal relationships may decrease libido and interfere with the ability to achieve and maintain an erection. Erectile dysfunction is reported in 50% of men with diabetes mellitus. The basis of this impotence is usually an autonomic neuropathy. However, vascular insufficiency, antihypertensive medication, uremia and depression may contribute to the problem in diabetics. A history of repeated nocturnal erections is indicative of psychogenic impotence. Thus, a history of erections that occur nocturnally, during masturbation, or during foreplay or with other sexual partners eliminates significant neurologic, vascular or endocrine causes of impotence.

5. B

Total lymphocyte count and cell-mediated immunity are the two most common tests to evaluate an immune deficiency state. Anergy or impaired immunity is diagnosed if no response is noted to any of the skin tests, whereas a positive response (5 mm or more of induration) to one or more skin tests indicates normal lymphocyte activity.

6. D

Chronic lymphocyte leukemia (CLL) is a neoplasm characterized by accumulation of mature-appearing lymphocytes in blood and bone marrow; 95% of cases involve B lymphocytes; spleen and lymph nodes may be infiltrated; patients are usually over 50 years old. CLL is frequently an incidental finding on CBC. The complications include cytopenia, Coombs-positive hemolytic anemia, hypo-gammaglobulinemia, infection, evolution into lymphoma (Richter's syndrome). Many patients require no therapy; some may need therapy with alkylating agents, glucocorticoids,or immunoglobulin infusion.

7. B; 8.C

Causes of gynecomastia:

Drugs (amphetamines, androgens, chorionic gonadotropin, hydroxyzine, isoniazid, meprobamate, methyldopa, phenothiazynes, and reserpine)
Primary hypogonadism secondary to Leydig cell damage
- Testicular germ cell or Leydig cell tumors
- Feminizing adrenocortical, adenoma or carcinoma

Familiar gynecomastia

In familiar gynecomastia the breast tissue is inordinately sensitive to normal levels of circulating estrogens. It seems that circulating prolactin hormone (in hyperprolactinemia or prolactin (PRL)-secreting pituitary tumors stimulates breast glandular development through its mammotropic action. In addition, elevated levels of PRL may also diminish the peripheral actions of testosterone, which may result in an excessive estrogen effect on the breast that is not counteracted by androgens. Feminizing tumors of the adrenals or Leydig cells are associated with marked elevations of serum estradiol. Serum PRL and thyroid hormones should be measured to detect hyperprolactinemia and hyper or hypothyroidism. Phenothiazine should be discontinue in order to measure levels of PRL (induced increase in PRL). Chest-x-ray may detect metastatic disease or an hCG-secreting primary lung neoplasm. CT scans of the pituitary-hypothalamic region should be performed if hyperprolactinemia is present. There are not complications of gynecomastia except for psychologic damage from the cosmetic defect. These patients have a slightly increased risk of breast carcinoma.

9. A; 10.D

Iritis is the inflammation of the anterior segment of the middle coat (uvea) of the eye. Suppurative iritis is seen in trauma or spread of an infection from an adjacent area (paranasal sinus) or systemic infection (bacterial endocarditis). Visual is usually diminished. Non suppurative causes include viral kerato-conjunctivitis, corneal foreign body or abrasion, ultraviolet keratitis..etc. Systemic diseases include: ankylosing spondylitis, psoriatic arthritis, Reiter's syndrome, Behcet's syndrome, sarcoidosis, inflammatory bowel disease, and various chronic infections including syphilis, tuberculosis, toxoplasmosis, and histoplasmosis. Patients with non-suppurative iritis complaint of painful eye, photophobia, and decreased vision. Almost all of the idiopathic iritis resolve in 2-4 weeks and permanent scarring of the iris can impair the normal pupillary dilatation and visual acuity. Topical steroids and hemotropin are indicated.

11. B; 12.A; 13.B; 14.D

The chest x-ray shows apical fibrocaseous tuberculous disease. Pulmonary disease is the most frequent clinical presentation of TB disease. Secondary involvement of the adrenal gland causes hyponatremia with hyperkalemia (hypoaldosteronism). Tuberculosis is more common among debilitated and otherwise immunocompromised patients (alcoholics and AIDS patients). Diagnosis is established by culturing the organism. Positive fluochrome or acid-fast smears are presumptive evidence of active tuberculosis. Treatment requires hospitalization, patient education, antibiotics and respiratory isolation.

15. D; 16.B

As a preoperative evaluation, a chest x-ray, EKG, blood gases and some basic pulmonary function tests are indicated. Although an evaluation of arterial oxygen tension is very helpful, the major reason for obtaining preoperative blood gases is to determine whether CO2 retention is present. This indicates severe pulmonary dysfunction and the need for an elective operative procedure must be reevaluated. The ratio FEV-1/ Vital Capacity less than 45 % with a decreased FEV-1, slight decreased DLCO and an increased residual volume are characteristic of a severe obstruction of the airway.

17. C

Neurofibromatosis is a heterogenous autosomal dominant disorder with two clinical presentations: neurofibromatosis (NF) I and NF II. NF type I presents the characteristic pigmented skin lesions referred to the cafeau-lait spot, pigmented hamartomas of the iris called Lisch nodules, and neurofibromas of the skin. In addition, freckling commonly is seen in the axillae or other intertriginous areas in NF type I. The margins of cafe-au-lait spots may be smooth. Neurofibromas may be discrete or diffuse and are composed of various combinations of Schwann cells, fibroblasts, neurons, and vascular elements. NF type II, or central neurofibromatosis, is not associated with cafe-au-lait spots, Lisch nodules, or other peripheral manifestations. Children may have associated brain tumors. Bilateral acoustic neuromas are diagnostic.

18. C

Squamous cell carcinoma (SCC) arises in the epithelium and is common in the middle-aged and elderly population. They are most common in sun-exposed areas: scalp, backs of hands, and superior surface of the pinna; They arises in skin that has been damaged by thermal burns or chronic inflammation. It also occurs from epidermal diseases of unknown origin such as Bowen's disease. SCC are often separated into two major groups based on their malignant potential. Those arising in areas of prior radiation or thermal injury, chronic draining sinuses, chronic ulcers, and Bowen's disease are typically aggressive and have a high frequency of metastases. SCC originating in actinically damaged skin are less aggressive and less likely to metastasize.

19. C

Habitual abortion is defined as 3 consecutive pregnancy wastage before 20 weeks gestation with a fetus weighing less than 500 g. In about 66% the cause is a genetic error (trisomy, polyploidy, and X monosomy), anatomic abnormalities of the reproductive tract (cervical incompetence, congenital uterine abnormalities, submucous leiomyomas, Asherman's syndrome), hormonal abnormalities (thyroid dysfunction, progesterone insufficiency, and diabetes mellitus), infection (Mycoplasma, Ureaplasma urealyticum, Toxoplasma gondii, Listeria monocytogenes, Neisseria gonorrhea, Chlamydia, herpes simplex, Treponema pallidum, Brucella), immunologic factors, or systemic disease (chronic hypertensive or chronic renal failure and collagen vascular diseases). In the other 33%, the cause is unknown.

20. A; 21.A; 22. D

Hypertrophic obstructive cardiomyopathy (HOCM) presents a marked LV hypertrophy; often asymmetrical, without underlying cause. Systolic function is normal; increased LV stiffness results in elevated diastolic filling pressures. Symptoms are secondary to elevated diastolic pressure, dynamic LV outflow obstruction, and arrhythmias. Dyspnea on exertion, angina, presyncope and sudden death may occur. Findings in the physical examination include a brisk carotid upstroke with pulsus bisferiens, S4, a harsh systolic murmur along left sternal border, a blowing murmur of mitral regurgitation at the apex. Murmurs change with Valsalva and other maneuvers. EKG shows LV hypertrophy with prominent «septal» Q waves in leads I, aVL, V5-6. Periods of atrial fibrillation or ventricular tachycardia are often detected by Holter monitor. Echocardiogram shows LV hypertrophy, asymmetrical septal hypertrophy, LV contractile function excellent with small end systolic volume. If LV outflow tract obstruction is present, systolic anterior motion (SAM) of mitral valve and midsystolic partial closure of aortic valve are present. The treatment is based in beta blockers, verapamil, or disopyramide to reduce symptoms. Digoxin, positive inotropic drugs, diuretics, and vasodilators are contraindicated. Endocarditis antibiotic prophylaxis is necessary when outflow obstruction or mitral regurgitation is present. Strenuous exercise should be avoided.

23. A

Auer rods are sharply outlined, red staining rods found in the cytoplasm in blast cells in the blood smear of patients with acute myelogenous leukemia.

24. D

Eosinophilia is present in patients with asthma, Loffler's syndrome, fibroplastic eosinophilia, and parasitic infections. Myxedema is associated with basophilia.

25. B

Early manifestation of malignancy with compression of the spinal cord is the onset of pain, localized in the area of nerve compression and in its dermatome. In case of new onset of back pain, patients known to have malignancy must be studied immediately.

26. A

Patients who present signs of spinal cord compression (pain, urinary incontinence, leg weakness...etc) should start dexamethasone i.v. immediately followed by radiation therapy. Laminectomy with spinal cord decompression is indicated in some cases (e.g. lymphoma). In any case, the initial treatment must be i.v. dexamethasone.

27. D

Superior vena cava obstruction syndrome (SVCS) is most commonly caused by cancers that arise in or spread to the mediastinum, such as lymphoma or lung cancer. The presence of a mass by chest radiograph or CT scan usually confirms the diagnosis. Histologic diagnostic can be obtained via bronchoscopy or mediastinoscopy. Myelography is not a procedure of choice in these patients.

28. B

Breast cancer causes hypercalcemia in 30-40% of the cases followed by multiple myeloma (20-40%), lung (12-35%), head and neck (2.9-3.5%) and renal cell carcinoma (<1.5%).

29. C

Hemolytic anemia is characterized by an increased destruction of red blood cells that can occur because of an intrinsic (cell membrane or enzymatic) defect in the red blood cell, an extrinsic (extracorpuscular) abnormality, or an abnormality in hemoglobin or globin synthesis. Common extrinsic abnormalities include hypersplenism, certain drugs, antibodies directed at red blood cells, and mechanical damage. Combinations of these forms may also occur. Abnormalities common to all types of anemia in this category are elevated serum bilirubin and LDH, depressed serum haptoglobin, and reticulocytosis (polychromatophilic macrocytes or nucleated red blood cells) on the peripheral blood smear.

30. D

Neonatal risk in neonates of diabetic mothers are: respiratory distress syndrome, hypoglycemia, poor feeding, hypocalcemia and hyperbilirubinemia.

31. D

Most common side effects of benzodiazepines are: drowsiness, dizziness, fatigue, and incoordination. They can cause paradoxic agitation more marked in geriatric population, delirium, falling, respiratory depression with a variety of deleterious effects on psychomotor performance and cognitive side effects like reduction in the ability to learn new information (anterograde amnesia). Discontinue the administration of chronic high doses of benzodiazepines can produce a severe withdrawal syndrome include delirium and grand-mal seizures.

32. B; 33.B

The diagnosis of esophageal atresia with tracheoesophageal fistula can be made when a nasogastric tube fails to pass into the stomach. Chest-x-ray reveals the tube coiled in a blind esophageal paunch. Treatment include constant suction of the esophagus, 30oC elevation of the head to prevent reflux of gastric contents into the lung and preparation for surgical repair.

34. B

Strokes occurring as a complication of myocardial infarct are usually caused by emboli arising from left ventricular thrombi. Aspirin can prevent the thrombi formation and strike a small percentage of patients.

35. C

Small thoracic cage usually is seen in the chest-x-ray.

36. C

Lead poisoning. Sources of lead are: Paint soil, household dust, drinking water and several types of industries. Clinical presentations in childhood include : Abdominal pain irritability, lethargy, anorexia, pallor (anemia), ataxia, slurred speech, seizure, coma, death (associated with pica and malnutrition). Subclinical: mental retardation language and cognitive deficits behavior abnormalities. In adults may present headache, abdominal pain, anemia, renal disease, peripheral neuropathy, ataxia, memory loss, encephalopathy, wrist drop or food drop.

37. D; 38.B; 39.C; 40.A

Marfan's syndrome. Disorder of the connective tissue resulting in long, thin limbs, scoliosis, pectus excavatum, hypermobile joints. Tay-Sachs disease. Autosomal recessive disorder seen most frequently among ashkenazi jewish. Phenylketonuria. Most common amino acid disorder due to a deficiency of a hydroxylase enzyme. Dietary restriction can avoid the mental retardation. Galactosemia. Inborn error of carbohydrate metabolism. After milk feedings the infants present hepatomegaly, vomiting, amino aciduria, and growth failure.

41. B

Other complications of acute sinusitis include: brain abscess, epidural empyema and sagittal sinus thrombosis. Acute sinusitis can cause local expansion complications (orbital cellulitis, orbital abscess, sinus abscess and osteomyelitis).

42. C

Alport's syndrome is a disease usually in males in the second decade of life. It may present with hematuria, hypertension and deafness, but not mental retardation.

43. E

Antipsychotic medications and its side effects.
(see table C.1)

44. B; 45.D

Patients with tardive dyskinesia (TD) present lateral jaw movements and «fly-catching» motions of the tongue. A prolonged holiday from neuroleptics may cause the symptoms to diminish or disappear within 3 months. However, in many individuals, dyskinesia is irreversible and persists after discontinuation of therapy. TD is postulated to result from an increased number of dopamine receptors that are synthesized in response to long-term dopamine receptor blockage. This makes the neuron supersensitive to the actions of dopamine and allows the dopaminergic input to this structure to overpower the cholinergic input, causing excess movement in the patient.

46. A

The most frequent cause is adenovirus. This double-stranded linear DNA virus causes a variety of diseases such as upper respiratory tract infections such as pharyngitis, pharyngo-conjunctival fever, and acute respiratory disease manifest with varying degrees of fever, sore throat, coryza, and conjunctivitis. In the lower respiratory tract, atypical pneumonia is characterized primarily by fever, cough, and patchy consolidation. Hematuria and dysuria are prominent in hemorrhagic cystitis. Gastroenteritis with nonbloody diarrhea occurs mainly in children under two years of age. Most adenovirus infections resolve spontaneously. Approximately half of all adenovirus infections are asymptomatic.

47. D

Pneumothorax, empyema and purpura with disseminated intravascular coagulation is a clinical picture caused by Staphylococcus infection.

48. E

Improper feeding is the most common cause of acute diarrhea in early infancy. There is wide variation in tolerance among infants to both the quality and quantity of food. Throughout infancy and childhood, infections are the most common causes of diarrhea. These include both infectious diarrheas as well as certain infections outside the Gl tract that are frequendy associated with diarrhea in infants. In contrast to infants with diarrhea from improper feeding, infants with infectious causes of diarrhea appear ill; there may be fever and m some, CNS signs, depending on the causative agent. In temperate dimates human rotavirus is responsible for 50% of all diarrheal illness and up to 80% of cases of severe diarrhea in infants in winter. Parvovirus-like agents have been associated with major outbreaks of acute diarrhea in Norwalk, Connecticut, Hawaii, and Montgomery County, Maryland. Bacterial pathogens probably cause 10 to 15% of acute diarrheal disease in children . The most commonly identified pathogens in children in North America are Campylobacter jejuni, strains of Salmonella and Shigella, and Yersinia enterocolitica. Although E. coli is a. Parasitic agents, including Entamoeba histolytica and Giardia lamblia, produce diarrhea; toddlers, particularly those in day-care centers, commonly acquire giardiasis.

49. D

The nephrotic syndrome is characterized by proteinuria, hypoproteinemia, edema and hyperlipidemia. Most of the children with nephrosis (90%) have some form of the idiopathic nephrotic syndrome of unknown etiology. Minimal-change disease (85%), mesangial proliferative (5%) and focal sclerosis (10%) are histologic findings of this syndrome.

50. C

Table C.1

Table C.1: **Antipsychotic medications and its side effects.**

Effects	Sedative	Hypotensive	Extrapyramidal
Chlorpromazine	+++	+++	++
Thioridazine	+++	+++	+
Fluphenazine	+	+	+++
Trifluoperazine	+	+	+++

Vitamin D deficiency appears as rickets in children and as osteomalacia in postpubertal adolescents. The pathophysiology of rickets results from defective bone growth, especially marked at the epiphyseal cartilage matrix, which fails to mineralize. The uncalcified osteoid results in a wide, irregular zone of poorly supported tissue, the rachitic metaphysis. This soft, rather than hardened, zone produces many of the skeletal deformities through compression and lateral bulging or flaring of the ends of bones. The clinical manifestationi of rickets are most common during the first 2 years of life and require several months of a vitamin D-deficient diet to become evident. Craniotabes is due to thinning of the outer table of the skull, which feels to the touch like a Ping-Pong ball when compressed. Enlargement of the costochondral junction (rachitic rosary) and thickening of the wrists and ankles may be palpated. The serum calcium usually is normal but may be low, the serum phosphorus level always is reduced, and the serum alkaline phosphatase activity is elevated.

51. A

The most frequent cause of hemolytic anemia in neonate is fetal erythroblastosis characterized by: (1) the maternal Rh-negativity and presence of antibodies on indirect Coombs' test, (2) Rh or other antibody titer, (3) history of previous infant with hemolytic disease of the newborn and (5) postnatal fetal cord blood findings of Rh-positivity and anemia (hemoglobin < 10 g).

52. A; 53.D; 54.E (see figure C.42)

Fractures of the skull are probably among the most important injuries to diagnose in the trauma setting. They are classified as closed or open and nondepressed or depressed. Closed fractures have no associated break in the overlying soft tissues. Open fractures allow the meninges to communicate with the outside and include injuries that communicate with the sinuses. Both of these situations carry a significant risk of meningitis. Depressed fractures are those in which bone has been displaced below the normal margin of the calvarium. Often, these fractures should be suspected of having produced intracranial injury, and CT should be performed in most situations. Fractures of the temporal bone are often associated with epidural hematomas because of

Table C.2: **Spinal fluid findings in disease**

Disease	Appearance	Cells/mm3	Protein (mg/dL)	Glucose (mg/dL)	Other
Tuberculous meningitis	Opalescent faintly yellow; fibrin clot	50 to 300; monos	60 to 700	< 20	Positive for acid-fast bacilli
Fungal and yeast meningitis	Opalescent	30 to 500; monos	100 to 700	< 30	Serology for Cryptococcus positive
Acute purulent meningitis	Turbid	Few to 20,000; chiefly polys	100 to 700	< 20	Positive smear
Viral meningitis and encephalitis	Clear, colorless	Few to 350; chiefly monos	40 to 100	N	Virus cultures may be positive
Brain abscess	Clear, colorless may be xanthochromic	Few to 100; monos predominate	40 to 140	N	Negative cultures
Early subarachnoid hemorrhage	Bloody; faintly yellow	Many RBCs	50 to 400	N	
Late subarachnoid hemorrhage	Slightly bloody; supernatant deep yellow	Fewer RBCs; WBCs increase due to aseptic meningitis	100 to 800	May be depressed	RBC's dissapear in 2 weeks. S

N = Normal
Monos = Monocytes
RBC = Red blood cells
WBC = White blood cells

Table C.2

rupture of the middle meningeal artery. Secondary signs of trauma in the sinuses may indicate significant intracranial pathology. The most important is an air-fluid level in the sphenoid sinus seen on the brow-up lateral film that is often associated with a basilar skull fracture. In this situation, cerebrospinal fluid leaks into the sphenoid sinus, causing the air-fluid level. If a skull fracture communicates with the sphenoid, ethmoid, or posterior wall of the frontal sinuses, it is classified as «open» and needs antibiotic coverage because of the possibility of infection.

55. A

Listeria monocytogenes is found in a wide variety of habitats, including milk and milk products (both unpasteurized and pasteurized) and in plants and vegetables. High risk of developing listeriosis are pregnant women and their fetuses, newborn infants, debilitated elderly persons, and immune compromised hosts. Septicemia and meningitis can be developed. Rare cases of purulent conjunctivitis, lymphadenitis, abscesses, endocarditis, peritonitis, arthritis, pneumonitis and cholecystitis are been reported. Usually patients with listeriosis should be treated with penicillin or ampicillin and an aminoglycoside for at least 3 months in order to avoid relapses.

56. B

Occasionally other symptoms such as nocturnal or morning cough, halitosis, reduced sense of smell, or diminished vocal resonance may suggest sinus infection.

Figure C.42

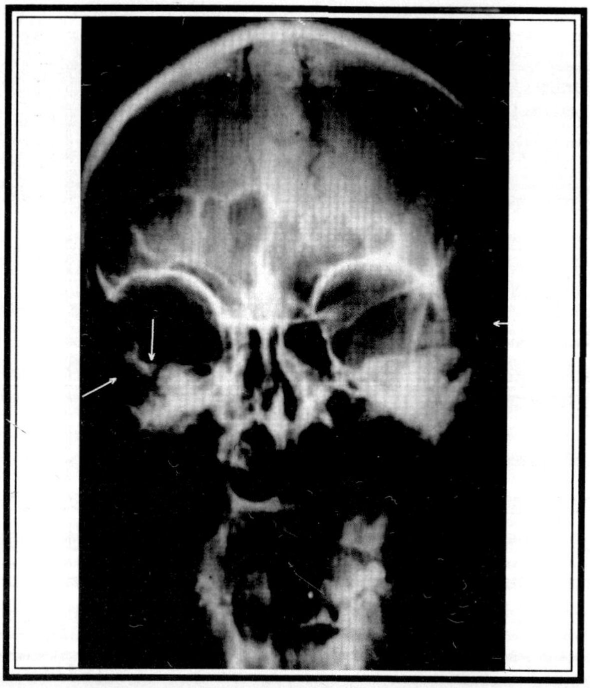

57. E; 58.C; 59.A; 60.B; 61.A

Spinal fluid findings in disease (see table C.2)

62. C; 63.A; 64.C

Reperfusion arrhythmias (ventricular tachycardia and PVCs) are commonly seen in patient during the thrombolysis. Several mechanisms have been involved in the production of these arrhythmias included the formation of oxygen metabolites. The treatment of VT or frequent PVCs is lidocaine in bolus followed by an i.v. infusion (2-4 mg/minute).

65. A; 66.D; 67.B; 68.C; 69.D

Grand mal seizures. It is usually idiopathic with typical sequence of tonic-clonic events and postictal effects. Absence seizures. It is abrupt onset of seizures with no postictal effects. It should be treated with ethosuximide. Partial complex seizures. It presents a sudden onset of unresponsiveness with staring and postictal effects. Automatisms are seen during the period of unresponsiveness. Treatment usually includes phenytoin and/ or tegretol. Pseudoseizures. This seizure disorder usually requires no anticonvulsivant therapy. It is often gradual, presenting bizarre actions and behavior with no evidences of biting or incontinence.

70. B

Hypoglycemia is the most common postoperative complication and most often follows the use of long-acting insulin given subcutaneously before surgery. Blood glucose levels should be measured every 2-4 hours and the patient monitored for signs and symptoms of hypoglycemia (eg, anxiety, tremulousness, and profuse sweating without fever).

71. E; 72.C; 73.C; 74.D

Breathing room air, the ABG's show a significant A-a gradient. This gradient does not improved breathing 100 percent oxygen suggesting a large right-to-left shunt. Alveolar ventilation (VA) is increased, as evidenced by a low arterial PCO2. A spinal tap is not indicated at present. Cyanotic congenital heart disease is the most likely choice, as demonstrated by the cyanosis, low arterial PO2 breathing 100% oxygen, and the deepening of cyanosis on crying. The absence of a murmur and normal ECG are not unusual with congenital heart disease, especially in the first day of life. His tongue is dusky, indicating central cyanosis. Oxygen given by mechanical ventilation is not indicated since no beneficial effect was demonstrated on blood gas determination. Cardiac catheterization and cineangiography should be carried out as soon as possible. Life-threatening congenital cardiac defects require prompt surgical therapy. Tetralogy of Fallot is rarely seen in the immediate newborn period. The lack of a murmur over the pulmonary area rules against this diagnosis. The low pressure in the left ventricle and the high oxygen saturation in the pulmonary artery are against tetralogy of Fallot. Transposition of the great vessels is the leading type of serious cyanotic heart disease in the newborn period. Cyanosis, tachypnea, and increased pulmonary vascularity are all features of transposition. Normal heart size and lack of a murmur in the first 24 hours of life are not unusual. Treatment consists in balloon septostomy.

75. C

Patients with adrenal insufficiency undergoing the stress of operation are at risk of addisonian crisis manifested by salt wastage, decreased blood volume, hypotension, shock and death. For at least 2-3 days preoperatively, they should receive fluid and sodium chloride replacement intravenously (usually 1-3 l/day) and cortisol therapy (20 mg each morning and 10 mg each afternoon). On the day of surgery, they should receive 100 mg of cortisol intramuscular or intravenous just before the operation, followed by 50-100 mg every 6 hours during surgery.

76. B

A number of DNA and RNA-containing retrovirus are oncogenic. They are able to induce malignant transformation of cultured cells. The viral genome is usually integrated into the DNA of the host cell. Transformed cells lose normal growth control mechanism. Oncogenes are present in normal cells and may be activated by virus infection.

77. D; 78.D; 79.E; 80.E

Impetigo is a common contagious, superficial skin infection, which is produced by streptococci, staphylococci, or a combination of both bacteria. Symptoms of itching and soreness are mild. Impetigo may occur after a minor skin injury. The disease is self limiting, but when untreated it may last for weeks or months. Poststreptococcal glomerulonephritis may follow impetigo. Rheumatic fever has not been reported as a complication of impetigo. ASO titer elevations are low or absent, but anti-DNAase B and antihyaluronidase increase significantly. Total serum complement activity is low during initial stages of acute nephritis. The C3 level correlates with the total serum complement. Sedimentation rate correlates with the activity of the disease. Cultures of the pharynx and any skin lesion should be made and the serotype of group A streptococcus responsible should be determined. Serotypes associated with acute nephritis are 2, 49, 55, 57, and 60. Acute nephritis heals without therapeutic intervention. Prevention. Triple antibiotic ointments containing bacitracin, polysporin, and neomycin should be applied three times daily to sites of minor skin trauma. Local therapy such as mechanical debridement of crusts, washing with antibacterial soaps, and applying antibacterial creams are beneficial. Infected children should be briefly isolated until treatment is under way. The oral or parenteral administration of antibiotics results in a higher and more predictable cure rate. Although the efficacy of systemic antibiotics in preventing acute nephritis has not been conclusively demonstrated. Because most cases of impetigo have a mixed infection of staphylococci and streptococci, penicillin is no longer the drug of choice. A 10-day course of the appropriate oral dosage of cloxacillin, dicloxacillin, or cephalexin will induce rapid healing.

81. C; 82.E; 83.C; 84.A

Primary adrenocortical insufficiency or Addison's disease in 20% of the cases is secondary to TB infection. Eighty percent of the cases is associated to an autoimmune endocrine disorder. Other less common disorders include adrenal hemorrhage and infarction, fungal infection, metastatic and lymphomatous replacement, amyloidosis, sarcoidosis, hemochromatosis, radiation therapy, cytotoxic agents (mitotane), enzyme inhibitors (metyrapone), surgical adrenalectomy,...etc. Calcification of the adrenals is almost pathognomonic of TB. Symptoms are fatigue, weakness, anorexia, hypotension and hypoglycemia. Mineralocorticoid deficiency produces renal sodium wasting and potassium retention with dehydration and acidosis. Treatment include administration of glucocorticoids and correction of hydration (volemia and electrolytes). Cortisol (hydrocortisone) is most commonly used. Patients with primary Addison's disease and electrolyte abnormalities may need an additional mineralocorticoid agent (fludrocortisone).

85. A

Idiopathic Addison's disease is frequently accompanied by gonadal failure, hyperthyroidism, hypothyroidism, Hashimoto's thyroiditis, diabetes mellitus, vitiligo, hypoparathyroidism, and pernicious anemia. The association of any of these endocrine disorders with Addison's disease is called Schmidt's syndrome.

86. A

Patients with hyperthyroidism must become euthyroid before surgery. This takes 1 to 6 weeks and is best accomplished by treatment with propylthiouracil. If emergency surgery is required, adequate sedation and potassium iodide plus a adrenergic blocking agent such as propranolol should be given in addition to propylthiouracil.

87. A

The substantial growth in health care expenditures is based in an increase average age of the American population, advances in technology and the adoption of Medicare and Medicaid to the health system.

88. B; 89.C

Acetazolamide. It is a weak diuretic inhibitor of carbonic anhydrase which inhibits the exchange of H+ for Na+ in proximal convoluted tubule.

Furosemide. It inhibits the Na+/K+/Cl- co-transport in ascending loop of Henle resulting in retention of Na+, Cl- and water in the tubule.

90. C

The locked-in syndrome (pseudocoma) describes patients who are awake but selectively deefferented, i.e., have no means of producing speech or limb, face, or pharyngeal movements. This results from infarction or hemorrhage of the ventral pons, which transects all descending corticospinal and corticobulbar pathways but spares the RAS arousal system. Vertical eye movements and lid elevation are partially preserved because these midbrain functions are outside the field of infarction in some cases of basilar artery thrombosis. Such movements can be used by the patient to signal to the examiner.

91. B

Malabsorption in patients with chronic pancreatitis. A fecal fat concentration in excess of 10% is characteristic of chronic pancreatitis as a cause of steatorrhea. The D-xylose test is positive in the presence of small bowel disease and usually is normal in patients with pancreatic exocrine insufficiency. The secretion stimulation test becomes abnormal when more than 75% of pancreatic function is lost. Normally, the peak concentration of bicarbonate in pancreatic juice is greater than 80 mEq/L. Patients with abdominal pain secondary to chronic pancreatitis who do not have steatorrhea have concentrations in the range of 60 to 80 mEq/L. Diarrhea is frequently but not invariably associated with pancreatogenous steatorrhea. Stools typically are soft, greasy, and foul-smelling. An oily ring is left in the toilet bowl. Most patients with steatorrhea respond to replacement of pancreatic enzymes. If this fails to reduce fecal fat excretion to less than 15 to 20 g/day, fat content in the diet should be decreased. If steatorrhea persists, aluminum-containing antacids, and finally, cimetidine are introduced. The Schilling test for vitamin B12 absorption shows decreased urinary secretion of labeled cyanocobalamin in 40% of patients with chronic pancreatitis but may also be positive in the presence of pernicious anemia, bacterial overgrowth, or ileal disease.

92. C

Portal hypertension. Portal hypertension is an elevation in pressure of the portal venous circulation (normal pressure ranges from 7 to 10 mm Hg). The average portal pressure in these patients is 20 mm Hg with a range of 15 to 60 mm Hg. Mechanisms of portal hypertension are: (1) increased resistance to portal blood flow and (2) increased portal blood flow. Alcoholic cirrhosis causes obstruction of portal venous blood flow on the hepatic vein side of the sinusoid (postsinusoidal). The most common cause of portal hypertension is cirrhosis of the liver, most frequently caused by chronic alcoholism. Laennec's cirrhosis accounts for 85% of cases of portal hypertension in the U.S. In children, extrahepatic portal venous occlusion is the most common cause of portal hypertension. This is most commonly a consequence of cavernomatous malformation of the portal vein.

93. D

There are no evidences that estrogens can induce carcinoma from normal breast tissue. Oral contraceptive users have a lower incidence of nonmalignant breast disease. There appears to be no increased risk of endometrial cancer. A reported increased risk of dysplasia among oral contraceptive users does not necessarily consider other factors such as multiplicity of sexual partners, early onset of sexual activity, and the use of other methods of contraception. An increase in hepatocellular adenoma, has been reported in oral contraceptive users. These tumors are benign but may induce significant morbidity, when rupture (hemorrhage).

94. C

* The Child's classification is an additive clinical and laboratory parameters to determine the liver and nutritional status. Those who are Child's class A are good-risk patients with low operative mortality. Those in Child's class C are high-risk patients with correspondingly higher operative mortality (see table C.3).

Table C.3

Table C.3: **CHILD'S CLASSIFICATION**

	A	B	C
Serum bilirubin (mg/dl)	Below 2.0	2.0-3.0	Over 3.0
Serum albumin (mg/dl)	Over 3.5	3.0-3.5	Under 3.0
Ascites	None	Minimal	Advanced
Neurologic disorder	None	Easily controlled	Poorly controlled
Nutrition	Excellent	Good	Poor

USMLE step 3

ANSWERS

BOOKLET C TEST 2

1. C

Sexual drive usually increases with the intake of small amount of alcohol and is inhibited after the intake of large amounts of alcohol. Sexual activity is inhibited in diabetics due to an organic etiology (frequently vascular-atherosclerotic disease).

2. C; 3.D; 4.A; 5.D

The most common cause of penile ulcerations are herpes simplex virus (HSV). Primary infection causes painful grouped vesicles on an erythematous base. The vesicles then ulcerate in the first week, crust in the second week and heal without scarring. Recurrent HSV infection (type II) recurs a mean of 4 times a year. Diagnosis is based in clinical finding and viral cultures. Treatment requires acyclovir 200 mg 5 times/day for 10 days. Recurrent HSV infections can be treated with acyclovir 200 mg 2-5 times/day for several days (5 days). Pregnant women with active genital lesions at the time of delivery should be delivered by cesarean section to reduce the likelihood of transmission to the neonate. Acyclovir has not been approved for use in pregnancy.

6. B; 7.A

The EKG shows a run of ventricular tachycardia. VT is frequent after myocardial ischemia and they are life-threatening conditions. The electrocardiographic diagnosis criteria are: QRS duration of 140 ms or more, left axis deviation, fusion and capture beats, AV dissociation, and QS morphology in V5 or V6. Ventricular tachycardia usually presents with bizarre QRS morphology, though it can simulate either a left or right bundle branch block. The availability of a prior EKG is helpful. Emergency DC countershock should be used in patients presenting in an unconscious state without a palpable pulse. In patients who present with a pulse and hypotension, cardioversion may be accomplished with synchronized DC countershock. Subsequently, intravenous lidocaine should be started to prevent recurrent attacks until the patient has stabilized. In hemodynamically stable patients, lidocaine in bolus and i.v. infusion is the treatment of choice.

8. D

Methylxanthines have a weak diuretic action resulting in an increased urinary output of sodium, chloride, and potassium.

9. E

Hypothyroid patients are subject to acute hypotension, shock and hypothermia during surgery. If the patient is allowed to breathe spontaneously, severe CO2 retention may result from hypoventilation. Myxedema coma should be suspected in patients who fail to awake promptly from anesthesia and who manifest CO2 retention and hypothermia.

10. D; 11.E; 12.C

Chronic pain, somatization, multiple or vague physical complains, and preoccupation with the physical symptoms of depression are common chief complains of depressed patients. Fatigue, multiple unexplained complaints, and sleep disturbance are frequent. This patient suffers of stress-induced somatization process induced by severe and unusual psychosocial stressors. The underlying disease is a major depression with recurrent death thoughts, worthlessness, decreased interest, concentration and memory impair, appetite change, sleep change, fatigue and low energy. The treatment of major depression is primarily pharmacologic (doxepin, nortriptyline...etc). Full-dose therapy for 4-6 weeks is needed before therapeutic response can be assessed reliably. Supportive psychotherapy usually is appropriate for all depressed patient and can provided by the primary care practitioner. Most patients with depressive disorders can be managed by the primary care practitioner.

13. E

Cardiac disease may be exacerbated by many of the physiologic changes accompanying surgery, including fluctuations in heart rate, blood pressure, blood volume, oxygenation, pH and coagulability. These conditions may lead to myocardial ischemia due to increased myocardial demand or reduced coronary blood flow, impaired myocardial contractility, and altered cardiac performance due to changes in preload or afterload.

14. C

DM type I is associated with a deficient insulin secretion, they often present an immune-mediated destruction of the pancreatic beta cells and they are most likely to develop ketoacidosis if exogenous insulin is withheld. Type II DM may develop hyperosmolar coma. The percentage of glycosilated hemoglobin in blood reflects the blood glucose levels over a period of 2-3 months before the current measurement. Obesity is characterized by decreased in number or affinity of insulin receptors.

15. C; 16.D; 17.A

Mycoplasma pneumoniae causes «atypical» pneumonia. It is a pathogen only for humans. In the lungs, the organism is rod-shaped, with a tapered tip that contains specific proteins which serve as the point of attachment to the respiratory epithelium. During M. pneumoniae infection, autoantibodies are produced against red cells (cold agglutinins) and brain, lung, and liver cells. These antibodies may be the source of the extrapulmonary manifestations of infection. This organism is the most frequent cause of pneumonia in young adults and is responsible for outbreaks in groups with close contacts such as families, military personnel, and college students. The onset of M. pneumonia infection is gradual, usually beginning with a nonproductive cough, sore throat, or earache. Small amounts of whitish, nonbloody sputum are produced. Constitutional symptoms of fever, headache, malaise, and myalgias are pronounced. The paucity of findings in the physical examination is in marked contrast to the prominence of the chest x-ray infiltrates.

18. E

A stiff neçk or meningismus associated with headache is usually seen in patients with deep neck abscesses, cervical osteomyelitis, brain abscess and complicated sinusitis. The headache of meningeal irritation (infection or hemorrhage) is acute in onset, severe, generalized, deep-seated, constant, especially intense at the base of the skull, and associated with stiffness of the neck on bending forward. Dilatation and congestion of inflamed meningeal vessels are probably the main cause of the pain.

19. B

About 20% of the general population have some type of migraine headache. The typical headache pattern of migraine is recurrent unilateral headache accompanied by nausea or vomiting, with symptom-free periods of days, weeks, or months between episodes. Common migraine lacks the discrete aura—typically visual spots, lines, or scotomas—that occurs a few minutes before classic migraine. Cluster headache occurs more commonly in men and is so named because of the tendency of headaches to occur in clusters. A cluster may extend over several weeks, during which time the patient is typically awakened by severe retro-orbital headache with unilateral tearing, rhinorrhea, flushing, and occasionally oculosympathetic paralysis. The headache lasts 30-90 minutes, usually recurs every night, and may be misdiagnosed as sinus headache because of its location or trigeminal neuralgia because of its intensity.

20. C; 21. D; 22. E

Aortic stenosis (AS) can be congenital, secondary to rheumatic inflammation or may be due to degenerative calcification of the aortic cups. A peak systolic gradient exceeding 50 mm Hg in the face of a normal cardiac output or an effective aortic orifice less than 0.5 cm2 per square meter of body surface area, is considered critical obstruction to left ventricular outflow. A large «a» wave in the left atrial pressure pulse is seen in severe AS. Cardiac output at rest can be normal and may fail to rise during exercise. Symptoms often appear in the fifth or seventh decades. Exercise dyspnea, angina and syncope are the three cardinal symptoms. Systolic ejection murmur which commences shortly after the first heart sound, increases in intensity to reach a peak toward the middle of the ejection period and diminishes progressively thereafter to end just before aortic valve closure. It is low-pitched, rough, and rasping and is loudest at the base of the heart, and transmitted to the jugular notch and upward along the carotid arteries. EKG and echocardiogram reveals left ventricular hypertrophy. The average duration of various symptoms in patients not treated surgically was as follows: angina pectoris, 3 years; syncope, 3 years; dyspnea, 2 years; and congestive heart failure, 1.5-2 years.

23. D

Approximately 85% of diabetics over age 50 years produce and secrete enough insulin therefore, they require only diet or sulfonylureas to control the glycemia. If the serum glucose level is below 250 mg/dL on the morning of surgery, sulfonylureas should be withheld and 5% glucose solution should be administered intravenously at a rate of about 100 ml/h. This means that over a 10-hour period, only 50 g of glucose would be given (diabetic patients in a regular day would consume four times this amount). During any but the most extensive surgery, the pancreas should be able to produce enough insulin to handle this modest glucose load and at the same time prevent undue gluconeogenesis. If the fasting glucose level is above 250-300 mg/dL or if the patient is taking small doses of insulin but does not actually require insulin to prevent ketoacidosis, an alternative approach would be to add 5 units of insulin directly to each liter of 5% glucose solution being given at 100 mL/h. If the operation is lengthy, blood glucose levels should be measured every 3 to 4 hours during surgery to ensure adequate glucose control. The goal is to maintain glucose levels between 100 and 200 mg/dl.

24. E; 25. E

Erythema Nodosum is characterized by the presence of painful red nodules on the anterior surfaces of the lower legs.
They are most frequently the response to infection (tuberculosis, streptococcus, cryptococcus..etc), antibiotics, sarcoidosis, pregnancy, inflammatory bowel diseases or contraceptives. Lesions represent a nonspecific hypersensitivity reaction. Aspirin is an unusual cause of E. nodosum.

26. C; 27.A; 28.B; 29.A

Complications of peptic ulcers include: (1) hemorrhage, (2) obstruction, and (3) perforation. Hemorrhage occurs in 15% of patients with duodenal ulcer. Most of them respond satisfactorily to medical treatment. Free perforation into peritoneal cavity occurs in 6% of patients with duodenal ulcer. A plain upright radiograph of the abdomen may show the presence of free air under the diaphragm. Those ulcers located posteriorly may penetrate into adjacent structures, most often the pancreas, with increased in activity of serum amylase. Gastric outlet obstruction occurs in 2-4% of patients with pyloric channel or duodenal ulcers. These patients have symptoms of bloating, nausea, vomiting, and weight loss, and usually have symptoms of ulcer and obstructive symptoms for several months. Dumping syndrome is a rapid gastric emptying of a large osmotic load, resulting in distention of the jejunum and subsequent excessive secretion of water and electrolytes into the intestinal lumen.

30. B

The administration of intravenous fluids should be careful avoiding to overload the circulation. Monitoring of intake, output, body weight, serum electrolytes and central venous pressure is important in evaluating cardiorenal response and tolerance in this age group. Anesthesia requires doses of strong narcotics and are frequently depressed by routine doses. Codeine is usually well tolerated. Sedative and hypnotic drugs often cause restlessness, mental confusion, and uncooperative behavior in the elderly and should be used cautiously. Preanesthetic medications should be limited to atropine or scopolamine in the debilitated elderly patient and anesthetic agents should be administered in minimal amounts.

31. B; 32.A; 33.C; 34.B; 35.A; 36.D

Prothrombin time is the clotting time measured after addition of tissue factor and phospholipids to recalcified plasma. Prolongation of this test also occurs in deficiencies of factor VII, V, X, prothrombin or fibrinogen (<100 mg/dl). Template bleeding time is prolonged in thrombocytopenia (<100,000/uL), qualitative platelet disorders and vascular disorders. It also may be abnormal in patients treated with aspirin-containing medications. Activated partial thromboplastin time depends of the intact intrinsic and common coagulation pathways. Ristocetin-induced platelet agglutination assesses the presence of plasmatic von Willebrand factor. Factor IX concentration in serum is measured in patients with hemophilia (type B).

37. A; 38.E; 39.D

Systemic lupus erythematosus (SLE) is an immunologically mediated disease of unknown etiology. The principal mechanism of injury is deposition of circulating immune complexes. DNA single and double stranded is a major antigenic component of immune complexes. Clinical findings include the malar (butterfly) rash or fixed erythematous rash, flat or raised, over the cheeks and bridge of the nose, often involving ears and chin. It is usually exacerbated by ultraviolet light. Hair loss, usually in patchy or extensive is common. Vasculitis skin lesions include subcutaneous nodules, ulcers, purpura and infarcts of skin or digits. Symmetric arthritis, myopathy, glomerulonephritis, mental dysfunction, seizures, psychosis, organic brain syndrome, headache meningitis, neuritis, thrombosis in vessels, anemia, pancytopenia, pericardial and pleural effusions, or retinal vasculitis with infarcts are other signs and symptoms of this disease. Stillbirths and spontaneous abortion are high and there may be an increased flares of SLE during the first trimester and during the 6 weeks after postpartum. Treatment requires non-steroidal antiinflammatory drugs, hydroxychloroquine in the subacute cutaneous lupus and photosensitivity, glucocorticoids in life-threatening disease, cyclophosphamide in patients refractory to non-steroidal antiinflammatory drugs and dialysis or kidney transplantation in terminal renal failure. Chronic leukemia is not a complication in the course of SLE or its treatment.

40. E

Many factors have been alleged to influence wound healing. However, only a few are of possible clinical significance. These include protein depletion, ascorbic acid deficiency, marked dehydration or edema, and severe anemia. It has been shown that hypovolemia, vasoconstriction, increased blood viscosity, and increased intravascular aggregation and erythrostasis resulting from remote trauma will interfere with wound healing by reducing tissue oxygen tension.

41. A; 42.B; 43.D; 44.D

Septicemia and shock septic result from acute invasion of the bloodstream by certain microorganism or their toxic products. Fevers, chills, tachycardia, tachypnea, and altered mentation are common acute manifestations of septicemia. When hypotension and inadequate perfusion develop, the condition is termed septic shock. Systemic vascular resistance decreases, myocardial contractibility is poor, and pooling and altered distribution of blood in the microcirculation is seen. Diffuse cell and tissue injury and ultimately, widespread organ failure develop. It is most commonly caused by gram negative bacteria (E. coli, Klebsiella-Enterobacter, Proteus, Pseudomonas, and Serratia) followed by staphylococci and pneumococci. Hemodynamic responses include decrease in systemic vascular resistance (SVR) and increase in cardiac output (CO), in contrast with cardiogenic or hypovolemic shock where SVR is high and CO is low. Progressive lactic acidosis secondary to poor tissue perfusion is associated with poor outcome. Initial hyperventilation and development of adult respiratory distress syndrome (ARDS) is common. Evidences of disseminated intravascular coagulation in septic shock is an ominous prognostic sign. Treatment include respiratory support (mechanical ventilation), hemodynamic support (intravenous colloid and/or crystalloid solutions, vasopressor drugs: dopamine with or without norepinephrine and dobutamine if the heart is not able to maintain an adequate cardiac output) search for the origin of infection and antibiotics.

45. C

This african B cell lymphoma has been strongly related to the Epstein-Barr virus infection. It presents as a primary extralymphatic african tumor arising from jawbones. Because the rapid proliferation of the malignant cells, this is a poor prognosis hematologic lymphoma.

46. B

Acute leukemias are known to appear after exposure to ionizing radiation and genetic predisposition. Lymphoblastic and myeloblastic types occur, the former primarily in children. The two types can be distinguished on morphological and immunochemical grounds. The diagnosis is usually obvious since the patients are so sick. They have granulocytopenia with infections, thrombocytopenia with hemorrhages, and anemia. Bone marrow pain, splenomegaly, and adenopathy are common. Peripheral blood smears show an abundance of blast cells with few mature polys, but the total WBC count can be very high (>100,000) or below normal. Cerebral hemorrhage is common, perhaps initiated by plugging of small vessels by rigid blast cells.

47. C

Infections in patients with granulocytopenia are the most common cause of fever as well as mortality. Because there are not enough granulocytes, the typical consolidation seen in the chest-x-ray is commonly not seen. Gram-negative bacteria are responsible for most pneumonias and bacteremias and they should be treated with a cephalosporin (3rd generation) plus an aminoglycoside. Chemotherapy should be stopped until infection is controlled and white count is improved

48. A; 49.A

Recurrent palpitations is a common presentation of atrial fibrillation (AF). Hypertension is one of the common causes of AF but other diseases such as hyperthyroidism, Wolf-Parkinson-White syndrome, ischemic heart disease, and valvular heart disease must be rule out. Intravenous digital is indicated in order to control the ventricular rate. After 3 weeks of anticoagulation, pharmacological or electrical cardioversion should be attempted.

50. C

Clinical criteria for diagnostic of Zollinger-Ellison syndrome are: (1) an increased in serum gastrin concentration, (2) increase in basal acid output, (3) an increased ratio of basal to peak (pentagastrin-stimulated) acid output, and (4) the presence of peptic ulcer disease or diarrhea or both, and a gastrin producing tumor. It occurs most frequently between ages 35-65 years in patients who complains of abdominal pain (ulcers), diarrhea and occasionally steatorrhea. Gastric mucosa is hypertrophic.

51. C

The most sensitive test to determine body iron stores is bone marrow iron stain.

52. B

Primary biliary cirrhosis is a disorder of unknown etiology, occurring most commonly in middle-aged females. It is characterized by a non-suppurative cholangitis, initially associated with a cholestatic syndrome and progressing over an extended period of years to cirrhosis and death due to complications. Characteristic features include an association with autoimmune disorders, and positive serum mitochondrial antibodies. Patients complain of pruritus and may develop xanthomas. Cholestyramine (Questran), 12-16 grams/day in divided doses, acts binding bile acids in the intestinal lumen, decreasing the bile acid accumulation in the skin, therefore alleviating the pruritus.

53. C

Hemochromatosis may be the most common autosomal recessive disease in humans. Symptoms of this disease include weight loss, weakness, fatigue, right upper quadrant abdominal pain, joint pain, excessive thirst and urination, palpitations, and impotence. The most common physical finding are gray-bronze pigmentation of the skin, hepatomegaly, enlargement and tenderness of the metacarpophalangeal joints and knees, decreased body hair, and testicular atrophy. In serum, transferrin saturation, iron concentration, serum ferritin concentration, glucose concentration and hepatocellular enzymes are all elevated. Plasma testosterone and dihydrotestosterone in men, or plasma estradiol in women are decreased.

54. B; 55.C; 56.B

Acute blood loss usually results in normochromic normocytic

anemia. Erythroid hyperplasia in the bone marrow, and an increase of the reticulocytes in the peripheral blood are common findings in hemorrhage and hemolysis in an attempt of bone marrow compensation.

57. C

This disorder results from a defect in hemoglobin structure. Traits occur in the heterozygous state along with normal adult hemoglobin, in a nonsymptomatic condition. The destruction of the red cells is mechanical and no immune-mediated. A single amino acid substitution (valine for leucine) in the beta-chain is the cause of this disease. At low pH and with decreased oxygen tension, HbS precipitates, the cells change its shape and vascular obstruction with hemolysis is seen.

58. D

Carcinoma of the colon and the rectum continues to be the most common cancer of the gastrointestinal tract. In men is the third most common cause, preceded only by cancer of lung and prostate. In women, it is outnumbered only by breast cancer. The peak of incidence is 80 years. Change in bowel habits and rectal bleeding may occur first. Symptoms of abdominal pain, bloating, constipation, and diarrhea are caused by partial bowel obstruction. Obstruction is móre common in carcinoma of the left colon, whereas carcinoma of the right and transverse colon frequently presents with weakness and anemia. Bleeding per rectum is a often finding, characterized by bright red or dark blood, with or without clots. Weight loss, and poor appetite are signs of advanced carcinoma. Septicemia and endocarditis caused by S. bovis is suggestive of carcinoma of the large bowel. Work up should include digital examination, barium enema, flexible sigmoidoscopy and colonoscopy. Carcino-embryonic antigen has been shown to have prognostic value.

59. B; 60.D

This patient has varicella or chickenpox. In the primary infection, the lesions are in various stages of development in different areas of the body. Primary infection occurs via the respiratory route and is followed by viremia. Reactivation results in herpes zoster infection. It is presumed that during chickenpox, the dorsal root ganglia are infected, and there the virus remains latent until reactivated. The incubation period ranges between 10 and 21 days. Patients are infectious 48 h before vesicles erupt, during vesicle formation and until all vesicles are crusted. The incidence of herpes zoster infection is highest in the sixth through eighth decades of life but can occur at any age. Low-grade fever and malaise may precede exanthem by 24-48 hours. Fever and lassitude generally last 3-5 days in immunocompetent hosts. The rash consists of maculopapules, vesicles, and scabs in various stages of evolution. Characteristic lesions are vesicles described as «dewdrops on a rose petal.» The most common complication of varicella is bacterial superinfection of the skin usually caused by Streptococcus pyogenes or Staphylococcus aureus. In children, CNS involvement consists of cerebellar ataxia and meningeal irritation, which generally occurs about 21 days after the onset of rash, is usually self-limited, and does not require hospitalization. Other CNS manifestations include aseptic meningitis, encephalitis, transverse myelitis, Guillain Barre syndrome, and Reye's syndrome. Varicella pneumonia is the most common serious complication of chickenpox occurring more commonly in adults (up to 20%). Other complications include myocarditis, corneal lesions, nephritis, arthritis, bleeding diatheses, acute glomerulonephritis, and hepatitis. The treatment of chickenpox in adolescents or adults is acyclovir for an infection of < 24 hours.

61. B

Hhigh output heart failure is seen in patients with hyrotoxicosis, beri-beri, systemic arteriovenous fistula and vascular shunts.

62. A

The eating behavior is controlled by the hypothalamus. Lesions in the ventromedial hypothalamus produce extreme obesity.

63. C; 64.B

The hallmark of a restrictive pattern is a decrease in lung volumes, primarily total lung capacity and vital capacity (FVC). In pulmonary parenchymal disease, residual volume is also generally decreased, and forced expiratory flow rates are preserved. In fact, when FEV-1 is considered as a percent of the FVC, the flow rates are often supranormal. This patient should quit smoking at least four days before surgery (recommended for both restrictive and obstructive disease).

65. C

Xanthomas are non-tender, firm, yellow to red papules and nodules. Location: elbows, knees, Achilles tendons related to genetic disorder of lipoprotein metabolism (primary) or secondary to an underlying disease (diabetes mellitus).

66. D

Complication of liver cirrhosis are portal hypertension, gastrointestinal hemorrhage, portosystemic encephalopathy, peptic ulcer disease and esophageal varices.

67. C

Enlargement of the spleen may occur in a great variety of circumstances. Most frequent is secondary to infectious diseases and malaria is still the most frequent etiology. The spleen may be markedly enlarged in parasitic infections, including leishmaniasis and hydatid disease. In portal hypertension it can be found considerable enlarged and may be accompanied of hypersplenism (anemia, thrombocytopenia, and leukemia). Increase in blood destruction (hemolytic anemia), excessive production of red cells (polycitemia), and in neoplastic proliferation (lymphomas, leukemia) the spleen can be involved and enlarged is often seen. Metabolic disturbances such as Gaucher's disease as well as a variety of granulomatous disease may lead to splenic enlargement. Immunological abnormalities (systemic lupus erythematous, rheumatoid arthritis), may also be accompanied by splenomegaly. Slightly enlarged spleen is seen subacute endocarditis and in rare cases of disseminated tuberculosis.

68. E

Urgency, precipitancy and frequency of micturition are common symptoms seen in patients with nervous system disease such as multiple sclerosis, bladder tumor, urinary infection, and cystitis.

69. E; 70.A; 71.B; 72.E; 73.E

Generalized crescentic glomerulonephritis (Idiopathic rapidly progressive glomerulonephritis) presents a marked extra-capillary (parietal epithelial) cell proliferation with crescent formation. It is more common in the elderly and affects equally males and females. Nearly all patients are admitted in renal failure with azotemia, oliguria, and, occasionally, anuria. They develop irreversible renal failure, leading to death within weeks or months. Complaints are usually nonspecific, consisting of sudden onset of nausea, vomiting, and weakness of several days duration. There is no history of antecedent infection. The ASO titer and serum complement are normal, cultures for pathogenic microorganisms are negative, and there is no evidence of involvement of organs other than the kidney. Renal arteriogram shows normal-sized or enlarged kidneys strongly suggestive of a recent acute process. Hypertension and edema may occur, but are rather uncommon. Corticosteroids and other immunosuppressive drugs have been found ineffective. In order to maintain life, permanent hemodialysis is necessary. By light microscopy, 80 to 90 percent of the glomeruli show florid epithelial crescents. Idiopathic crescentic glomerulonephritis must be differentiated from a variety of disease entities with similar clinical and pathologic features, such as Goodpasture's syndrome, fulminant poststreptococcal glomerulonephritis, progressive anaphylactoid purpura, and the microscopic form of polyarteritis nodosa. All of them may present with rapidly developing renal failure and epithelial crescents.

74. D; 75.C

Bargaining. Search for meaning in life and often by a return to religious institutions. This stage is marked by a belief that some magical power will intervene. Depression. Emotional detachment and a relinquishing of social and family bonds and responsibilities.

76. E

Indications for the PPD test include individuals with signs or symptoms of TB infection, recent contacts with known or suspected cases of tuberculosis, abnormal radiographic findings compatible with past tuberculosis, patients with diseases that increase the risk of tuberculosis (silicosis, gastrectomy, diabetes, immune suppression, HIV infection), and groups at high risk of recent infection with M. tuberculosis (immigrants, long-time residents and workers in hospitals, nursing homes, prisons, and inner city or skid-row populations).

77. D

Conversion disorder can be related directly to a psychological conflict and usually is not related to alcohol abuse.

78. D

Opiates dependency is suspected in those patients who complains of illnesses that require pain medication and who use multiple drugs prescribed by many physicians. Physicians have a feeling of being manipulated for patients who are usually of young age.

79. C

The smear shows a microcytc hypochromic anemia. Etiology. Iron deficiency anemia results from increased loss of iron (eg, occult gastrointestinal bleeding); or, occasionally, inadequate supply of iron (eg, malabsorption syndromes, subtotal gastrectomy, decreased intake); or increased demand for iron (eg, pregnancy).

80. D

In this tracing contractions are coming very frequently in the second stage of labor, consistent with abruptio placentae. With each contraction the fetus responds with variable decelerations which return promptly to baseline. The baseline seems to fluctuate between absent variability and average variability. The baseline variability is extraordinarily flat except where it is punctuated by the sawtooth pattern. The majority of the variable decelerations, irrespective of amplitude, are accompanied by small overshoot patterns. Although the baby spends most of its time decelerating, there is no real suggestion that the baseline heart rate is rising or that the fetal condition is deteriorating from the point of view of asphyxia. This tracing reflects significant neurologic abnormality.

81. C

Hyperkalemia usually occur when the serum potassium concentration is >6.5 mEq/liter. Cardiac manifestations include bradycardia that can progress to asystole, prolongation of atrioventricular (AV) conduction leading to complete heart block, and ventricular fibrillation. As the serum potassium increases, the EKG manifests progressive changes. Initially, peaked or tented T waves appear. Subsequently, ST segment depression, first-degree AV block, and QRS widening occur. Finally, a biphasic wave (sine wave) representing fusion of the widened QRS and T wave develops, signaling imminent ventricular standstill.

82. A

A cystometrogram involves filling the bladder to measure

volume-pressure relationships. As the bladder is filled to its normal capacity of 300-500 cc, the pressure inside the bladder should remain at less than 15 cm H2O. The patient usually experiences the first urge to void at 150-200 cc. In patients with GSI, the cystometrogram is normal. Patients with detrusor dyssynergia (DD) often have reduced bladder capacity and bladder contractions. The bladder contractions are demonstrated by a 15 cm H2O pressure increase above the baseline pressure.

83. A; 84. A

The EKG shows inverted T waves in lateral leads, compatible with myocardial ischemia. Although myocardial ischemia is more common in patients with diabetes mellitus, hypertension, hypercholesterolemia, smoking and obesity, toxins including cocaine ingestion or withdrawal of chronic exposure to nitroglycerin can cause sufficient coronary vasoconstriction to result in myocardial ischemia. Cocaine may also cause myocardial infarction.

85. C

Complete RBBB is characterized by prolonged QRS complex (0.12 second in duration) and an abnormal late portion of the QRS directed toward the right ventricle and away from the left ventricle. This is usually manifested by a broad terminal S wave in lead 1 and in other leads located over the left precordium such as V5 and V6, a terminal broad R wave in lead aVRI and the characteristic so-called RSR' complex in lead Vl. The right bundle is a relatively thin bundle of conduction fibers and is more vulnerable to interruption than the left bundle which branches early and widely. Thus RBBB may not imply myocardial damage as serious and as widespread as in block of the left bundle branch. RBBB may be caused by relatively small anatomic lesions although the most usual causes are idiopathic degenerative conduction system disease (causing fibrosis and interruption of the conduction fibers) and ischemic heart disease in the anterior septum where the right bundle courses.

86. D

In chronic pancreatitis. The classic syndrome consists of abdominal pain, diabetes, steatorrhea, and pancreatic calcifications. Chronic relapsing pancreatitis is characterized by intermittent pain without endocrine or exocrine insufficiency and calcification. In chronic pancreatitis, serum pancreatic isoamylase is usually normal or decreased. To treat the pain in chronic pancreatitis, alcohol and narcotics should be withdrawn (under cover of clonidine) if possible. The narcotic bowel syndrome may contribute to pain. Medically intractable pain suggests the need for surgery. The pain of chronic pancreatitis is severe and unremitting, usually causing drug addiction for analgesia.

87. B

Treatment of esophageal varices. Multiple large-bore intravenous lines and crossmatching of blood is the initial approach in patients with esophageal bleeding. Endoscopy is performed when the patient has become hemodynamically stable. If esophageal varices are identified as the source of bleeding, vasopressin, 0.4 to 0.8 units/minute, is administered by constant intravenous infusion. Patients who do not respond to vasopressin treatment require placement of the Sengstaken-Blakemore tube. Balloon tamponade will control variceal hemorrhage in most patients, but rebleeding rate is high once the balloons are deflated (50 to 60%). Sengstaken-Blakemore tube has the risks of perforation of the esophagus, necrosis of esophageal mucosa, and suffocation from migration of the balloon into the hypopharynx. Balloon tamponade is a temporary measure for control of bleeding, with up to 50 to 60% of patients rebleeding following balloon deflation. Acute variceal hemorrhage may be controlled with a single injection of a sclerosing agent in 70 to 80% of patients. Several (chronic) injections at weekly or monthly intervals is capable of obliterating esophageal varices. About half of patients treated by injection sclerotherapy will rebleed at some time. Injection sclerotherapy does not increase the overall survival in patients with bleeding esophageal varices.

88. E

Cholesterol intake averages about 450 mg per day in men and 300 mg in women. The important elements of the diet that primarily affect LDL cholesterol levels are saturated fat, cholesterol, caloric balance, and soluble fiber. The current intake of saturated fats is about 14% of calories. Monounsaturated fat (approximately 15% of calories) and polyunsaturated fats (approximately 7% of calories) do not elevate LDL cholesterol. Dietary cholesterol decreases the number of LDL receptors in the liver and causes an elevation in LDL concentrations. An overabundance of calories inappropriate to the person's physical activity level causes an increase im triglyceride synthesis by the liver with an increase in VLDL production rate. Obesity also increases free fatty acid flux to the liver. Soluble dietary fiber (eg, psyllium, guar, pectin) decreases LDL cholesterol probably by decreasing cholesterol absorption. Current guidelines for dietary modification to reduce cholesterol recommend a two-step approach. Step one: Reduction of saturated fat to less than 10% of calories, cholesterol to less than 300 mg/day and an increase in vegetable matter with more complex carbohydrates and additional fiber. Step two: Reduction of saturated fat to less than 7% calories, cholesterol to less than 200 mg/day and a further increase in complex carbohydrates.

89. D; 90.A; 91.C

Lower UTI is characterized by pyuria, often with dysuria, urgency, or frequency. A rapid, presumptive diagnosis can be made by microscopic examination of an unspun, clean-voided urine specimen. Urine collection under aseptic techniques often presents more than 103 bacteria/ml. Sites of infection in the genitourinary tract (e.g. epididymis prostate perinephric areas) are often associated with less than 103 bacteria/ml and have different clinical manifestations. Lower UTI usually occurs in women. Infections in men younger than 50 years of age are uncommon and suggest anatomic or functional abnormalities of the genitourinary tract. Men should have a complete genitourinary evaluation after their first infection; women should be evaluated after more than two recurrences within 1 year. Recurrent UTI may be associated with sexual activity. Chronic UTI is usually related to bladder instrumentation or catheterization or to significant urine residual produced by obstruction or neurogenic bladder dysfunction. The usual urinary pathogen in community-acquired UTI is Escherichia coli. Staphylococcus saprophyticus is a frequent pathogen in sexually active young women. Antibiotic therapy. Single-dose oral regimens are sufficient for symptomatic nonpregnant women with no known anatomic or functional abnormalities and no underlying illness. Regimens for 7-14 days are based on TMP/SMZ, amoxicillin, ampicillin or cephalexin. Adjunctive measures such as hydration and analgesia with phenazopyridine 200 mg PO tid may provide symptomatic relief during the first 24-48 hours. Failure of therapy for an infection due to a susceptible organism suggests an anatomic or functional genitourinary abnormality or persistent renal infection. Prophylaxis may be helpful for patients with frequent lower UTI. TMP/SMZ 40 mg/200 mg qd or qod is usually sufficient.

92. E; 93. A; 94. B; 95. B

Goodpasture syndrome is an anti-glomerular basal membrane (GBM) disease with lung and renal involvement. Diagnosis is based on either the presence of anti-GBM antibodies in the serum or the linear deposition of antibody along the basement membrane on renal biopsy. Anti-GBM disease is often rapidly progressive, requiring urgent diagnosis and treatment. Therapy may not be effective if the patient is already oliguric or receiving dialysis, or has a Creatinine greater than 6.5 mg/dl. The accepted therapeutic strategy in this disease is clearance of anti-GBM antibodies from the serum with concomitant suppression of formation of new antibodies. Plasmapheresis in combination with cyclophosphamide and prednisone over 8 weeks, may be effective.

USMLE step 3

ANSWERS

BOOKLET C TEST 3

1. C; 2. B

Most of the paroxysmal supreventricular tachycardias (PSVT) are produced by a reentry mechanism. Reentry has been localized to the sinus node, atrium, AV node, or to a macroreentrant circuit involving conduction in the antegrade direction through the AV node and retrograde through an AV bypass tract. Adenosine is the treatment of choice in this patient. This drug (6-12 mg i.v. bolus) may cause nausea, AV block and transient hypotension or atrial standstill. A complete work up for coronary artery disease is indicated.

3. B

Ulcerative colitis involves the rectum and spreads proximally.

4. C

Pericardial rubs are seen often in pericarditis with or without cardiac failure.

5. B

In acute leukemia, the neoplastic cells may infiltrate into the subarachnoid space, causing leukemic meningitis or direct involvement of the brain or spinal cord parenchyma. Neurologic involvement is unusual at the time of diagnosis, but the central nervous system is a frequent site of relapse, particularly in patients with ALL. The first symptoms of leukemic meningitis are usually headache and nausea. Papilledema, cranial nerve palsies, seizures, and altered mentation develop with disease progression. Cytocentrifuge preparations of cerebrospinal fluid (CSF) characteristically reveal leukemic blast cells, an elevated CSF protein, and reduced glucose concentrations.

6. D

Causes of hypercalcemia: (1) Parathyroid hormone-mediated: primary hyperparathyroidism, sporadic, familiar (multiple endocrine neoplasia types I and II), familiar hypocalciuric hypercalcemia, ectopic secretion of parathyroid hormone by tumors. (2) Non-Parathyroid hormone-mediated: malignant associated (local osteolytic hypercalcemia, humoral hypercalcemia of malignancy), vitamin D-mediated (intoxication with vitamin D, excessive production of 1,25(OH)D in granulomatosis disorders or sarcoidosis), other endocrinopathies (thyrotoxicosis, hypoadrenalism), immobilization with increase of bone turnover (Paget's disease), acute renal failure with rhabdomyolysis, calcium carbonate ingestion (mil-alkali syndrome).

7. D

Hyperosmolar coma is the result of severe dehydration. It may occur in undiagnosed diabetics who have been given large amounts of glucose during surgerical procedure. The resulting osmotic diuresis leads to disproportionate water loss, dehydration, and hyperosmolarity. Hyperosmolar coma is rarely seen until the serum glucose level exceeds 800 mg/dl and the osmolarity exceeds 340 mEq/l. Hyperosmolar coma may be best avoided by monitoring fluid input and output, measuring blood glucose levels, and instituting treatment promptly if the value exceeds 400 mg/dl.

8. A

Initial treatment of patients with tetanus is: (1) Wound management. Careful wound debridement and removal of necrotic tissue and foreign bodies are essential to remove the nidus of Infection and its toxins. (2.) Human tetanus immune globulin should be administered at a dose of 3000-6000 units intramuscularly to neutralize toxin not already fixed in the nervous system. (3) Penicillin G. 10 million units intravenously daily for 10 days. Supportive management should be: place the patient in an intensive care unit, in a quiet area with dim lighting until spasms, seizures, and autonomic instability (wide swings in blood pressure) have abated, as well as, sedation (diazepam), muscle relaxants (sometimes is necessary a neuromuscular blockade, which requires use of a ventilator and subjects the patient to the risk of pneumonia, atelectasis, or respiratory arrest if the patient is disconnected from the ventilator, control of seizures (phenobarbital), respiratory management, monitoring autonomic instability an nutrition.

9. B

Blockade of alpha-adrenergic receptors reduces the sympathetic tone of the blood vessels decreasing the peripheral vascular resistance. This induces reflex tachycardia.

10. C

Glutethimide and barbiturates have the highest risk for addiction liability and severe withdrawal symptoms.

11. B

The patient's EKG diagnosis is atrial flutter (AF) with variable A-V block. It usually occurs in patients with ischemic heart disease, rheumatic heart disease, or cardiomyopathy. It may also be seen in association with thyrotoxicosis, alcoholism, or pericarditis. The atrial rate is usually 250-350 beats/min. Treatment: (a) Carotid sinus massage. This maneuver may help make the diagnosis of atrial flutter by increasing AV block, thereby slowing the ventricular rate and uncovering flutter waves. (b) Pharmacologic cardioversion. In patients who are hemodynamically stable, loading doses of digitalis may be given to slow the ventricular response; subsequently, quinidine can be started to restore sinus rhythm. Propranolol or verapamil may be added to slow the ventricular rate transiently by producing a higher degree of AV block; however, these drugs do not affect the underlying atrial arrhythmia. (c) Rapid atrial pacing. If atrial flutter is unresponsive to drug therapy, atrial pacing may be utilized. If the patient is hemodynamically unstable, atrial flutter responds to synchronous DC cardioversion using low energies (25-50 J).

12. E

Chronic myelogenous leukemia (CML) is usually characterized by splenomegaly and production of increased numbers of granulocytes; course is initially indolent but eventuates in leukemic phase (blast crisis) rate of progression to blast crisis is variable, overall survival averages 4 to 5 years from diagnosis. More than 95% of patients have characteristic chromosomal abnormality, Philadelphia chromosome, with the formation of a fusion gene called bcr-abl. Blastic phase may involve cells of either Iymphoid or myeloid origin. Treatment of chronic phase involves control of cell counts with alkylating agents or hydroxyurea.

13. E; 14.A

The chest-x-ray shows a consolidation in the left lower lobe. The Gram stain shows abundant Gram-positive diplococci consistent with S. pneumoniae. HIV patients are at risk of having recurrent pneumonias, most of them community acquired. Once the lymphocyte count drops below 200/uL the probability of having opportunistic infections dramatically increases. In this case, penicillin is the antibiotic of choice.

15. D

Primary amenorrhea is the absence of menses by age of 16. It is seen in (see table C.4).

16. B

Puberty is considered precocious if menarche and secondary sexual characteristics occur before the age 9.

17. A

A low parathohormone (PTH) level is seen in malignancy. In primary hyperthyroidism PTH is elevated.

Table C.4: **Causes of primary amenorrhea**

	Causes
Genetic/development	Masculinization at puberty and in genetic disease (46,XX and 46,XY karyotype)
Physiologic	Pregnancy, puerperium and menopause
Failure of uterine response	Hysterectomy, cryptomenorrhea (stenosis of cervix or vagina), destruction of endometrium (Asherman's syndrome)
Ovarian insufficiency	Destruction (surgery, irradiation, infections), neoplasms, premature menopause, polycystic ovary (Stein-Leventhal) syndrome
CNS disorders	Pituitary hypothalamic dysfunction, tumors, steroid hormones
Endocrinologic	Thyroid disease, adrenal disease
Nutritional	Anorexia nervosa, malnutrition, morbid obesity
Others	Chronic systemic disease, psychogenic and psychotropic drugs

Table C.4

18. C

Peutz-Jeghers syndrome presents several maculas and spots of pigmentation around the mouth, as well as, intestinal polyposis.

19. D

Adolescence brings a cognitive view of death and a clear understanding of its irreversibility.

20. B; 21.D; 22.B; 23.C

Herpes zoster Infection is characterized by a unilateral vesicular eruption within a dermatome accompanied by severe local pain. Pain is the heralding symptom of infection and may precede the development of lesions by 48-72 hours. Lesions are erythematous maculopapules that evolve rapidly into vesicles. The most debilitating consequence of herpes zoster infection is acute neuritis and postherpetic neuralgia both more common in adults but the latter more common with advancing age. CNS involvement includes asymptomatic CSF pleocytosis, symptomatic meningoencephalitis with headache, fever, photophobia, meningitis, and vomiting, and rarely granulomatous angiitis with contralateral hemiplegia. Transverse myelitis with or without paralysis also may be seen. In immunocompromised patients, especially patients with Hodgkin's and non-Hodgkin's lymphoma, the clinical syndrome is more severe, and there is a greater risk for disseminated skin lesions or even visceral dissemination. Cutaneous dissemination occurs in about 40% of these patients. Visceral dissemination, including pneumonitis, meningoencephalitis, and hepatitis, occurs in 5-10% of patients with cutaneous dissemination.

24. C

The diffusion capacity of the lung is reduced in restrictive lung disease due to the thickening of the alveolar walls and the loss of the capillary bed (fibrosis).

25. A

Measurements of ventilatory function consists of quantification of the air contained within the lungs under certain circumstances and the rate at which air can be expelled from the lungs. Total lung capacity (TLC) is the volume of gas contained within the lungs after a maximal inspiration, while the residual volume (RV) is the volume of gas remaining within the lungs at the end of a maximal expiration. The volume of gas that is exhaled from the lungs in going from TLC to RV is called the vital capacity (VC).

26. A

Fluid volume of the pleural cavity may increase in presence of lymphatic obstruction or in patients with an elevated capillary hydrostatic pressure.

27. D

Beta-1 receptors are located in the myocardium and their stimulation cause positive inotropic and chronotropic responses. Beta-2 receptors are located throughout the body and their stimulation lead to reactions such as bronchodilation and vasodilation.

28. D; 29.C; 30.A

External otitis. Pain or itching of the ear canal with inflamed canal and normal tympanic membrane. Acute otitis media. Painful ear with strong evidence of inflamed tympanic membrane. Serous otitis media. «Blocked» painless ear with canal clear and dull immobile tympanic membrane.

31. D

Meconium aspiration syndrome is associated with placental insufficiency, cord disorders, hypertension, and fetal anoxia.

32. D

Hydramnios is an excessive quantity of amniotic fluid (more than 2,000 ml). By 36 weeks of pregnancy, the normal volume of amniotic fluid is approximately 1,000 ml. Incidence of hydramnios is high in diabetes erythroblastosis and twin pregnancies. Fetal malformations, particularly CNS and gastrointestinal tract defects, are often associated with hydramnios. Half of the cases of anencephalus and almost all cases of esophageal atresia are accompanied by hydramnios.

33. D

Bromocryptine is used for induction of ovulation in infertile female, to correct the luteal phase.

34. B

Anergy is associated with an increased susceptibility to infectious complications. Patients at high risk for immune deficiency include elderly patients and those with malnutrition, severe trauma, burns or cancer. Other than for a course of preoperative hyperalimentation, no stimulants of the immune system are consistently being used in the preoperative period.

35. C

GSI incontinence is caused by the loss of the normal anatomic angle between the bladder and the urethra. The angle loss allows the pressure inside the bladder to exceed the intraurethral pressure, resulting in the immediate loss of urine. GSI accounts for 75-80% of all cases of incontinence. Common causes of GSI include vaginal delivery, instrumented deliveries, and delivery of large infants. GSI is often associated with other pelvic relaxation problems, such as cystocele, rectocele, and uterine prolapse.

36. E

DD, unstable bladder or urge incontinence may be caused by uninhibited bladder contractions (motor urge incontinence) or strong sensory input from the bladder secondary to inflammation, tumors, or lack of estrogen (sensory urge incontinence). The patient has a sudden inability to control her bladder followed by a delayed loss of urine. In some patients, DD is caused by an upper motor neuron disease, such as multiple sclerosis. DD may also occur following pelvic surgery. The exact mechanism is unknown but is believed to be secondary to partial denervation of the bladder.

37. D

Serum bilirubin greater than 1.8 mg/dl, emesis of or intestinal malabsorption of the dye, inadequate hepatic excretion due to liver disease, or failure of the patient to take the pills can give a false-positive oral chelecystogram.

38. E

There is not clinical evidences that this patient is having and acute myocardial event. The EKG reveals deep Q waves in D2, D3 and AVF that suggests and old inferior MI. In the same EKG mild intraventricular conduction defects are seen.

39. A; 40.D; 41.D

42. A

Henoch-Schonlein purpura is characterized by non-thrombocytopenic leukocytoclastic vasculitic purpura, chiefly on the lower extremities and buttocks; abdominal pain, melena, hematochezia, and arthralgias. Acute renal failure occurs in up to 25% of adults. The skin lesions evolve from urticarial papules into the classic leukocytoclastic vasculitic lesions within 48 hours. The lesions are 2 to 10 mm in diameter and appear in crops among coalescent ecchymoses and pinpoint petechiae. Lesions fade in several days.

43. B; 44.E

The chest-ray shows significant cardiomegaly (dilated cardiomyopathy), with redistribution of the blood flow, secondary to congestive heart failure. Treatment includes to remove precipitating factors, digoxin, diuretics, venodilators (nitrates) and ACE-inhibitors (most important pharmacological interventions). Once the ejection fraction is less than 30% oral anticoagulation may prevent thromboembolism. Verapamil is not indicated in this patient due to the low ejection fraction.

45. D; 46.A; 47.B; 48.C; 49.E; 50.B

Hyponatremia is seen in patients with SIADH. Hypercalcemia should be suspected in patients with anorexia, nausea, thirst, polyuria, polydipsia, headaches, constipation, mood changes and shortened QT interval in the EKG. It is seen in malignancy with metastatic spreading and in excess of parathohormone. Hypomagnesemia is a frequent electrolyte abnormality seen in alcoholic intoxication and in patients treated with chemotherapy (cisplatinum, etoposide). Hypernatremia is most commonly seen with severe dehydration. Hyperkalemia is seen in patients treated with spironolactone, capoten or in renal failure.

51. B; 52. B; 53. D

A rapid enlargement of the thyroid gland and stridor can evolved in completed tracheal obstruction and death for asphyxia. Symptoms of this patient are manifestations of primary hypothyroidism confirmed with high levels of TSH and low thyroid hormones in serum. In addition, elevated level of thyroglobulin and thyroid microsomal antibodies is compatible with the diagnosis of Hashimoto's thyroiditis or chronic lymphocytic thyroiditis. A pulmonary flow-volume loop study shows evidence of upper-airway obstruction (variable extrathoracic obstruction as seen in the shortening and flattening of the inspiratory loop), and CT scan is useful in evaluating the obstruction and size of the infiltrating mass. Iodine uptake scans shows low radioactive uptake (5% in 24 hrs; normal values are <25% in 24 hrs) due to hypothyroidism. Treatment should include replacement with levothyroxine hormone (because inhibited of TSH, the uptake of the thyroid gland is also inhibited). Lymphoma is most likely to develop in the course of Hashimoto's thyroiditis. Because of the acute disease (upper airway obstruction) surgical intervention with partial thyroidectomy and release of the obstruction is indicated. According the histologic type (sections obtained from biopsies), extension of the lymphoma, and complications (upper airway obstruction) treatment with aggressive chemotherapy may be indicated.

54. C

Anti-cholinergic drugs cause tachycardia, dry mouth, blurring of vision, constipation, restlessness, confusion, and delirium.

55. C

Reactions that lead to generation of the prothrombin activator complex are: 1) by exposing plasma to a negatively charged surface such as glass or certain diatomacious earth powders (intrinsic pathway) or 2) by adding a lipoprotein activity from tissues called tissue factor to plasma (extrinsic pathway). In the intrinsic pathway, factor XII, prekallikrein, and factor XI come down onto a negatively charged surface where they react to give rise to activated factor XI. Factor XIa then activates factor IX. An intrinsic factor X activator the forms as a complex of the enzyme, factor IXa, an 2 cofactor, factor VIIIa and procoagulant phospholipid, present on the surface of activated platelet or of tissue cells. In the extrinsic pathway adding tissue factor to plasma provides a cofactor for factor VII. A factor VII/tissue factor complex initiates activation of factor X. The first factor Xa formed back-activates factor VII and the resultant factor VIIa/tissue factor complex becomes a many-fold more efficient activator of factor X. In the prothrombin time (PT), plasma is clotted with an unphysiological high concentration of tissue factor. Then, the factor VIIa/tissue factor complex directly activates factor X so rapidly that its indirect activation through an initial activation of factor IX becomes unimportant.

56. E

Complications of PTCA are: coronary artery dissection, occlusion of coronary arteries, CVA, spasm of coronary arteries and 5-10% can develop an acute myocardial infarct during the procedure. Those patients require an emergent CABG (coronary artery bypass).

57. D

Several radionuclide imaging techniques are of value in the diagnosis or assessment of myocardial infarction. Acute infarct scintigraphy is carried out with an infarct-avid imaging agent such as 99Tc stannous pyrophosphate. Scans are usually positive 2 to 5 days after infarction. Myocardial perfusion with Thallium 201, which is taken up and concentrated by viable myocardium, reveals a defect (cold spot) in most patients during the first few hours after development of transmural infarct. Radionuclide ventriculography with 99Tc-labeled red blood cells frequently demonstrates wall motion disorders and reduction in ventricular ejection fraction in patients with acute myocardial infarction. This tests is not indicated in AF.

58. D

With GSI, the patient often reports loss of urine with physical activity. These activities include coughing, sneezing, climbing stairs, laughing, bouncing, and intercourse. Urine loss is instantaneous and is often described as a «squirt» of urine. This is opposed to detrusor dyssynergia, in which urgency follows physical activity or occurs while at rest. The urge is then followed by a large loss of urine.

59. E; 60.B; 61.D

Porphyria Cutanea Tarda. It is the most common type of porphyria; characterized by chronic skin lesions and hepatic disease. It is due to deficiency of uroporphyrinogen decarboxylase. Photosensitivity causes enhanced facial pigmentation, increased fragility of skin, erythema, vesicular and ulcerative lesions, typically involving face, forehead, and forearms. Liver disease and hepatic siderosis may be related to alcoholism. Diabetes mellitus, SLE, and other autoimmune diseases may coexist. Urine uroporphyrin and coproporphyrin are increased. Abstinence from alcohol leads to improvement, and decrease in hepatic iron may ameliorate skin lesions. Chloroquine may be used in patients unable to undergo phlebotomy. Colicky abdominal pain, fever, leukocytosis, vomiting, constipation, port-wine colored urine, and neurologic and psychiatric disturbances are typical features of the intermittent acute porphyria.

62. C

Primary squamous cell carcinomas usually occur in the upper and midesophagus, and are more prevalent in persons with a history of significant alcohol intake and in smokers. Tumors in the distal third of the esophagus are more likely to be adenocarcinomas occurring at the gastroesophageal junction or in the location of a Barrett's esophagus.

63. E

Typical symptoms of reflux esophagitis include: frequent substernal burning discomfort after meals or at night occasionally associated with regurgitation of gastric juice is typical. Pain is relieved by sitting up. Severe disease can cause dysphagia because of stricture.

64. B

Elective mutism is a non-organic mental disorder characterized by voluntary refusal to speak seen in the infancy, childhood or adolescence. Idiosyncratic intoxication, uncomplicated alcohol withdrawal and withdrawal delirium, alcohol hallucinosis, alcohol amnestic disorder (Korsakoff's syndrome) and alcohol dementia (Wernicke's syndrome) are alcohol-induced organic mental disorders.

65. D

Pathogenic mechanisms of community acquired pneumonias include: aspiration, hematogenous spreading (Staphylococcus aureus), and inhalation of an infectious aerosol (TB, C. psittassi, C. burnetti and Influenza virus).

66. A; 67.B

Atrial fibrillation (AF) may be either chronic usually associated with organic heart disease due to coronary artery disease or mitral valve disease, or chronic obstructive pulmonary disease or paroxysmal, which may be seen with preexcitation syndromes, pulmonary embolism, thyrotoxicosis, and alcohol ingestion and, on occasion, without a demonstrable etiology. EKG shows an absence of atrial activity, and the ventricular response is usually an irregularly irregular rate between 160 and 200 beats/minute in the absence of AV node blocking drugs (digoxin, beta antagonists, verapamil). Therapy. Emergent cardioversion is necessary in patients with a rapid ventricular response and those who have angina, hypotension, dyspnea, or heart failure. In hemodynamically stable patients, digoxin, verapamil, propranolol, or esmolol can be given intravenously or orally to slow the ventricular response. Elective restoration to sinus rhythm can be attempted pharmacologically and should generally be done in a monitored hospital setting (procainamide, quinidine, or cardioversion). The patient should receive a 3-week course of oral anticoagulation before conversion and for 2-3 weeks after conversion.

68. B; 69.A; 70.C

Paralytic ileus is an absence of bowel sounds in patients after a recent operation with prolonged return of bowel function. KUB shows both small and large bowel gas without differential air/fluid levels. Mesenteric vascular occlusion is seen in elderly patients with recent MI who present sudden, severe abdominal pain an abdominal tenderness out of proportion to physical findings. Laboratory tests show: markedly elevated WBC count, hyperamylasemia, unexplained, persistent metabolic acidosis. Large bowel obstruction presents marked abdominal distention before significant symptoms appear. KUB shows distended gas-filled colon.

71. A

A diet high in fiber (bran, cellulose, etc.) appears to reduce the risk of diverticulitis.

72. D

Enteroenteral fistulas, abscess, and intestinal obstruction are the most common indications for small intestinal and ileocolic types. Perianal disease and medical failure as well as ileocolic fistulas and abscess formation are the most common indications for surgery in the colonic type.

73. C; 74. D; 75. B

The EKG shows an old inferior MI and significant changes in the anterior wall compatible with ischemia and injury. The positive enzyme pattern for MI and the clinical findings diagnostic of a subendocardial infarction. Diltiazem given within 72 hours of this type of infarction may prevent later reinfarction and recurrent angina in patients with non-Q-wave myocardial infarction; however, it may increase mortality in patients with Q-wave myocardial infarction and depressed left ventricular function. Most patients with non-Q-wave myocardial infarction are at risk for later events. By producing coronary vasodilatation and decreasing myocardial oxygen demand, calcium channel blockers may be beneficial in treating postinfarction angina.

76. D

Pheochromocytoma is characterized by labile severe hypertension, paroxysmal hypertension, a feeling of nervousness, headaches, palpitations, and a generalized appearance of hypermetabolism. There may be a recent onset of abnormal glucose tolerance.

77. A

Cushing's syndrome is suggested by obesity, typically distributed to the trunk and face. There may be striae. Weakness and muscle wasting are characteristic. There may be amenorrhea in women and impotence in men. Radiographic findings of osteoporosis are common. Back pain is frequent and pathology fractures of the vertebral bodies are seen.

78. B

Clubbing is a selective bullous enlargement of the distal segment of the digits due to an increase in soft tissue. It may be hereditary, or acquired. Acquired clubbing are associated with cyanotic heart disease, infective endocarditis, pulmonary disorders (such as: interstitial lung disease, carcinoma, bronchiectasis, lung abscess), gastrointestinal disorders (regional enteritis, chronic ulcerative colitis, and hepatic cirrhosis).

79. D

Surgical drainage is clearly indicated in subphrenic abscess, bacterial peritonitis and purulent pericarditis. Fibroexudative pulmonary tuberculosis is not a surgical indication and treatment is based in on multiple antibiotics given for at least 6 months .

80. D; 81.B

Ventricular tachycardia occurs most often in the setting of ischemic heart disease, acute myocardial infarction and classic or variant angina, following recovery of heart attack and in patients who develop ventricular aneurysm. Other causes include cardiomyopathy, prolonged QT syndrome, drug toxicity, and metabolic disorders. EKG shows widc QRS complexes (>0.12 sec) of abnormal morphology, occurring at a rate of 100-250 beats/minute and accompanied of ST- and T -wave changes in a direction opposite to the major QRS deflection. Treatment in stable patients requires i.v. lidocaine (bolus 1 mg/Kg), followed by continuous infusion of 2 mg/min. As a second choice, procainamide should be given. If patient is unstable (hypotension, heart failure, dyspnea or angina) immediate cardioversion is indicated.

82. D

Necrotizing soft tissue infections are serious conditions caused by clostridial and non-clostridial microorganism. These infections are marked by a layer of necrotic tissue, which is not walled off by a surrounding inflammatory reaction, and thus does not present a clear boundary. A clostridial infection classically involves underlying muscle, and is termed clostridial myonecrosis or gas gangrene. Most clostridial and non-clostridial infections spread in the subcutaneous fascia between the skin and the deep muscular fascia. Necrotizing fasciitis is the most common name for these infections. Cellulitis with ecchymoses, bullae, any dermal gangrene, or crepitus suggest an underlying necrotizing infection. Surgical intervention is critical step in this diagnosis. Non-clostridial infections is usually caused by S. pyogenes.

83. B; 84.A; 85.C; 86.C

The CT scan and the chest-x-ray show a mass in the right lung. Together with the clinical history, the most likely diagnosis is lung carcinoma. Lung cancers can be classified in: epidermoid (squamous), adenocarcinoma (including bronchioloalveolar), large cell, and small cell (including oat cells). Small cell is usually widely disseminated at presentation while non-small cell may be localized. Epidermoid and small cell typically present as central masses, while adenocarcinomas and large cell usually present as peripheral nodules or masses. Epidermoid and large cell may present central cavitation. Central endobronchial tumors cause cough, hemoptysis, wheeze, stridor, dyspnea, pneumonitis. Peripheral lesions can cause pain, cough, dyspnea, and symptoms of lung abscess. Extrathoracic metastatic disease affects 50% of patients with epidermoid cancer, 80% with adenocarcinoma and large cell, and over 95%

with small cell. Clinical problems result from brain metastases, pathologic fractures, liver invasion, and spinal cord compression. Endocrine syndromes include hypercalcemia (most often seen in epidermoid type), syndrome of inappropriate antidiuretic hormone secretion (small cell), gynecomastia (large cell). Skeletal connective tissue syndromes include clubbing in 30% (most often non-small cell) and hypertrophic pulmonary osteoarthropathy in 1-10% (most often adenocarcinomas), with clubbing, pain, and swelling.

87. D

Infective endocarditis usually occurs in an underlying valvular disease. The endothelium on the damaged valve leads to the formation of the vegetations at sites where a regurgitant jet of blood strikes. Glomerulonephritis is often seen (80% of the cases) and the vast majority of patients with tricuspid endocarditis develop pneumonia (or multiple septic emboli to the lungs).

88. C

Tetralogy of Fallot accounts for 6-15% of all cases of congenital heart diseases.

89. B

The signs of a small bowel obstruction are: mild to moderate, diffuse abdominal tenderness (severe, localized tenderness or signs of peritoneal irritation are indicative of complications, and may also indicate the cause of the obstruction); high-pitched, «tinkling» bowel sounds, an old abdominal scar, and abdominal distention which is generally a late finding.

90. D

The elasticity of the lung tissue is reduced. In addition, the area of gas exchange is reduced causing progressive dyspnea and hypoxemia.

91. C

Its half-life is 60-100 minutes and it is effective after 30-60 seconds of intravenous administration. It does not produce pharmacological effects in normal individuals and it has higher affinity for mu opiate receptors, reason why it is used to reverse the effects of heroin overdose.

92. D

Pulmonary congestion and pulmonary edema is seen in conditions that increase the capillary hydrostatic pressure (e.g. mitral stenosis).

93. B

M. pneumoniae (Eaton agent pneumonia) produces an influenza-like respiratory infection with gradual onset of headache, malaise, fever and non-productive cough. Physical findings are minimal despite extensive changes seen in chest-x-rays. Communicability of this agent is thought to be via large droplets of respiratory secretions; close indoor contact such as in household, institutional, or dormitory settings facilitates spread. Chest-x-ray most frequently reveals bronchial thickening with areas of interstitial infiltration and subsegmental atelectasis involving one of the lower lobes. «Platelike» atelectasis can be seen in lateral views. Leukocyte counts are often normal, but erythrocyte sedimentation is high and C-reactive proteins may be demonstrated. Fourfold elevation in sera titer of complement fixation test for M. pneumonia. Serology for cold hemagglutination must be obtained for the diagnosis of M. pneumoniae. Erythromycin and tetracycline derivatives are the treatment of choice.

94. D

Conditions that increase the cardiac work and oxygen demand can cause MI.Those conditions or factors are: increase in heart rate, hyperthyroidism and excess in catecholamines.

95. E; 96.C; 97.B

The CT scan and the chest-x-ray show an extensive pleural effusion with a mass in the left lung. In this case, the association of atelectasis (caused by the mass compressing the bronchial structures) and pleural effusion, make the trachea to stay in the central position. The proximity and invasion of the mass to the pericardium may cause pericardial effusion and tamponade The clinical findings are highly suspicious in this patient (lower extremities edema, jugulars engorged, hypotension). Lung cancers may present with cough, hemoptysis, wheeze, stridor, dyspnea, pneumonitis (central lesions). Peripheral lesions may cause pain, cough, dyspnea, symptoms of lung abscess resulting from cavitation.

98. E

Features of inflammatory bowel disease. Rectal bleeding is unusual in Crohn's disease but common in chronic ulcerative colitis. The findings of abdominal mass and anal complications (fissure, fistula) are more common in Crohn's disease. Terminal ileal involvement, skip areas, internal fistulas, and thumb printing are all rare or absent in chronic ulcerative colitis but common in Crohn's disease. Granulomas in the intestinal wall and adjacent lymph nodes are absent in ulcerative colitis but occur in 60% of patients with Crohn's disease. The colonic appearance of Crohn's disease is that of focal, predominantly right-sided disease. The mucosa is cobblestone in appearance with transverse ulcerations in affected areas. Biopsies reveal transmural disease with focal granulomas.

ANSWER SHEET

NAME (Please Print) ______ Last ______ First ______ Middle

TEST CENTER ______ CENTER NUMBER ______ DATE ______

SIGNATURE — REQUIRED FOR POSITIVE IDENTIFICATION OF ANSWER SHEET

ECFMG APPLICANT NUMBER GRID DIRECTIONS

Enter your ECFMG Applicant Number in the boxes to the left. Under each box blacken the circle that corresponds to the digit in that box.

0	0	0	0	0	0	0
1	1	1	1	1	1	1
2	2	2	2	2	2	2
3	3	3	3	3	3	3
4	4	4	4	4	4	4
5	5	5	5	5	5	5
6	6	6	6	6	6	6
7	7	7	7	7	7	7
8	8	8	8	8	8	8
9	9	9	9	9	9	9

DIRECTIONS:

- Use a black soft lead pencil (No. 2). DO NOT use a pen, a pencil with hard lead, or a pencil with liquid lead.
- Be sure to mark all answers on your answer sheet and completely fill the circle with a heavy, dark mark so that you cannot see the letter.
- Erase completely any answer you wish to change.
- Make no extra marks on this answer sheet.
- Mark only one answer for each question.

EXAMPLE

WRONG Ⓐ Ⓑ Ⓒ Ⓓ Ⓔ

WRONG Ⓐ Ⓑ Ⓒ Ⓓ Ⓔ

WRONG Ⓐ Ⓑ Ⓒ Ⓓ Ⓔ

RIGHT Ⓐ Ⓑ Ⓒ ● Ⓔ

COMPUTER USE ONLY

0	0	0	0	0
1	1	1	1	1
2	2	2	2	2
3	3	3	3	3
4	4	4	4	4
5	5	5	5	5
6	6	6	6	6
7	7	7	7	7
8	8	8	8	8
9	9	9	9	9

Test 1

1 Ⓐ Ⓑ Ⓒ Ⓓ Ⓔ	22 Ⓐ Ⓑ Ⓒ Ⓓ Ⓔ	43 Ⓐ Ⓑ Ⓒ Ⓓ Ⓔ	64 Ⓐ Ⓑ Ⓒ Ⓓ Ⓔ	85 Ⓐ Ⓑ Ⓒ Ⓓ Ⓔ
2 Ⓐ Ⓑ Ⓒ Ⓓ Ⓔ	23 Ⓐ Ⓑ Ⓒ Ⓓ Ⓔ	44 Ⓐ Ⓑ Ⓒ Ⓓ Ⓔ	65 Ⓐ Ⓑ Ⓒ Ⓓ Ⓔ	86 Ⓐ Ⓑ Ⓒ Ⓓ Ⓔ
3 Ⓐ Ⓑ Ⓒ Ⓓ Ⓔ	24 Ⓐ Ⓑ Ⓒ Ⓓ Ⓔ	45 Ⓐ Ⓑ Ⓒ Ⓓ Ⓔ	66 Ⓐ Ⓑ Ⓒ Ⓓ Ⓔ	87 Ⓐ Ⓑ Ⓒ Ⓓ Ⓔ
4 Ⓐ Ⓑ Ⓒ Ⓓ Ⓔ	25 Ⓐ Ⓑ Ⓒ Ⓓ Ⓔ	46 Ⓐ Ⓑ Ⓒ Ⓓ Ⓔ	67 Ⓐ Ⓑ Ⓒ Ⓓ Ⓔ	88 Ⓐ Ⓑ Ⓒ Ⓓ Ⓔ
5 Ⓐ Ⓑ Ⓒ Ⓓ Ⓔ	26 Ⓐ Ⓑ Ⓒ Ⓓ Ⓔ	47 Ⓐ Ⓑ Ⓒ Ⓓ Ⓔ	68 Ⓐ Ⓑ Ⓒ Ⓓ Ⓔ	89 Ⓐ Ⓑ Ⓒ Ⓓ Ⓔ
6 Ⓐ Ⓑ Ⓒ Ⓓ Ⓔ	27 Ⓐ Ⓑ Ⓒ Ⓓ Ⓔ	48 Ⓐ Ⓑ Ⓒ Ⓓ Ⓔ	69 Ⓐ Ⓑ Ⓒ Ⓓ Ⓔ	90 Ⓐ Ⓑ Ⓒ Ⓓ Ⓔ
7 Ⓐ Ⓑ Ⓒ Ⓓ Ⓔ	28 Ⓐ Ⓑ Ⓒ Ⓓ Ⓔ	49 Ⓐ Ⓑ Ⓒ Ⓓ Ⓔ	70 Ⓐ Ⓑ Ⓒ Ⓓ Ⓔ	91 Ⓐ Ⓑ Ⓒ Ⓓ Ⓔ
8 Ⓐ Ⓑ Ⓒ Ⓓ Ⓔ	29 Ⓐ Ⓑ Ⓒ Ⓓ Ⓔ	50 Ⓐ Ⓑ Ⓒ Ⓓ Ⓔ	71 Ⓐ Ⓑ Ⓒ Ⓓ Ⓔ	92 Ⓐ Ⓑ Ⓒ Ⓓ Ⓔ
9 Ⓐ Ⓑ Ⓒ Ⓓ Ⓔ	30 Ⓐ Ⓑ Ⓒ Ⓓ Ⓔ	51 Ⓐ Ⓑ Ⓒ Ⓓ Ⓔ	72 Ⓐ Ⓑ Ⓒ Ⓓ Ⓔ	93 Ⓐ Ⓑ Ⓒ Ⓓ Ⓔ
10 Ⓐ Ⓑ Ⓒ Ⓓ Ⓔ	31 Ⓐ Ⓑ Ⓒ Ⓓ Ⓔ	52 Ⓐ Ⓑ Ⓒ Ⓓ Ⓔ	73 Ⓐ Ⓑ Ⓒ Ⓓ Ⓔ	94 Ⓐ Ⓑ Ⓒ Ⓓ Ⓔ
11 Ⓐ Ⓑ Ⓒ Ⓓ Ⓔ	32 Ⓐ Ⓑ Ⓒ Ⓓ Ⓔ	53 Ⓐ Ⓑ Ⓒ Ⓓ Ⓔ	74 Ⓐ Ⓑ Ⓒ Ⓓ Ⓔ	95 Ⓐ Ⓑ Ⓒ Ⓓ Ⓔ
12 Ⓐ Ⓑ Ⓒ Ⓓ Ⓔ	33 Ⓐ Ⓑ Ⓒ Ⓓ Ⓔ	54 Ⓐ Ⓑ Ⓒ Ⓓ Ⓔ	75 Ⓐ Ⓑ Ⓒ Ⓓ Ⓔ	96 Ⓐ Ⓑ Ⓒ Ⓓ Ⓔ
13 Ⓐ Ⓑ Ⓒ Ⓓ Ⓔ	34 Ⓐ Ⓑ Ⓒ Ⓓ Ⓔ	55 Ⓐ Ⓑ Ⓒ Ⓓ Ⓔ	76 Ⓐ Ⓑ Ⓒ Ⓓ Ⓔ	97 Ⓐ Ⓑ Ⓒ Ⓓ Ⓔ
14 Ⓐ Ⓑ Ⓒ Ⓓ Ⓔ	35 Ⓐ Ⓑ Ⓒ Ⓓ Ⓔ	56 Ⓐ Ⓑ Ⓒ Ⓓ Ⓔ	77 Ⓐ Ⓑ Ⓒ Ⓓ Ⓔ	98 Ⓐ Ⓑ Ⓒ Ⓓ Ⓔ
15 Ⓐ Ⓑ Ⓒ Ⓓ Ⓔ	36 Ⓐ Ⓑ Ⓒ Ⓓ Ⓔ	57 Ⓐ Ⓑ Ⓒ Ⓓ Ⓔ	78 Ⓐ Ⓑ Ⓒ Ⓓ Ⓔ	99 Ⓐ Ⓑ Ⓒ Ⓓ Ⓔ
16 Ⓐ Ⓑ Ⓒ Ⓓ Ⓔ	37 Ⓐ Ⓑ Ⓒ Ⓓ Ⓔ	58 Ⓐ Ⓑ Ⓒ Ⓓ Ⓔ	79 Ⓐ Ⓑ Ⓒ Ⓓ Ⓔ	100 Ⓐ Ⓑ Ⓒ Ⓓ Ⓔ
17 Ⓐ Ⓑ Ⓒ Ⓓ Ⓔ	38 Ⓐ Ⓑ Ⓒ Ⓓ Ⓔ	59 Ⓐ Ⓑ Ⓒ Ⓓ Ⓔ	80 Ⓐ Ⓑ Ⓒ Ⓓ Ⓔ	101 Ⓐ Ⓑ Ⓒ Ⓓ Ⓔ
18 Ⓐ Ⓑ Ⓒ Ⓓ Ⓔ	39 Ⓐ Ⓑ Ⓒ Ⓓ Ⓔ	60 Ⓐ Ⓑ Ⓒ Ⓓ Ⓔ	81 Ⓐ Ⓑ Ⓒ Ⓓ Ⓔ	102 Ⓐ Ⓑ Ⓒ Ⓓ Ⓔ
19 Ⓐ Ⓑ Ⓒ Ⓓ Ⓔ	40 Ⓐ Ⓑ Ⓒ Ⓓ Ⓔ	61 Ⓐ Ⓑ Ⓒ Ⓓ Ⓔ	82 Ⓐ Ⓑ Ⓒ Ⓓ Ⓔ	103 Ⓐ Ⓑ Ⓒ Ⓓ Ⓔ
20 Ⓐ Ⓑ Ⓒ Ⓓ Ⓔ	41 Ⓐ Ⓑ Ⓒ Ⓓ Ⓔ	62 Ⓐ Ⓑ Ⓒ Ⓓ Ⓔ	83 Ⓐ Ⓑ Ⓒ Ⓓ Ⓔ	104 Ⓐ Ⓑ Ⓒ Ⓓ Ⓔ
21 Ⓐ Ⓑ Ⓒ Ⓓ Ⓔ	42 Ⓐ Ⓑ Ⓒ Ⓓ Ⓔ	63 Ⓐ Ⓑ Ⓒ Ⓓ Ⓔ	84 Ⓐ Ⓑ Ⓒ Ⓓ Ⓔ	105 Ⓐ Ⓑ Ⓒ Ⓓ Ⓔ

ANSWER SHEET

NAME (Please Print) ______________________________
Last First Middle

TEST CENTER ______________ CENTER NUMBER ______________ DATE ______________

SIGNATURE – REQUIRED FOR POSITIVE IDENTIFICATION OF ANSWER SHEET

ECFMG APPLICANT NUMBER GRID DIRECTIONS

Enter your ECFMG Applicant Number in the boxes to the left. Under each box blacken the circle that corresponds to the digit in that box.

DIRECTIONS:

- Use a black soft lead pencil (No. 2). DO NOT use a pen, a pencil with hard lead, or a pencil with liquid lead.
- Be sure to mark all answers on your answer sheet and completely fill the circle with a heavy, dark mark so that you cannot see the letter.
- Erase completely any answer you wish to change.
- Make no extra marks on this answer sheet.
- Mark only one answer for each question.

EXAMPLE

WRONG Ⓐ Ⓑ Ⓒ Ⓓ Ⓔ

WRONG Ⓐ Ⓑ Ⓒ Ⓓ Ⓔ

WRONG Ⓐ Ⓑ Ⓒ Ⓓ Ⓔ

RIGHT Ⓐ Ⓑ Ⓒ ● Ⓔ

0 1 2 3 4 5 6 7 8 9

COMPUTER USE ONLY

Test 2

1 Ⓐ Ⓑ Ⓒ Ⓓ Ⓔ	22 Ⓐ Ⓑ Ⓒ Ⓓ Ⓔ	43 Ⓐ Ⓑ Ⓒ Ⓓ Ⓔ	64 Ⓐ Ⓑ Ⓒ Ⓓ Ⓔ	85 Ⓐ Ⓑ Ⓒ Ⓓ Ⓔ
2 Ⓐ Ⓑ Ⓒ Ⓓ Ⓔ	23 Ⓐ Ⓑ Ⓒ Ⓓ Ⓔ	44 Ⓐ Ⓑ Ⓒ Ⓓ Ⓔ	65 Ⓐ Ⓑ Ⓒ Ⓓ Ⓔ	86 Ⓐ Ⓑ Ⓒ Ⓓ Ⓔ
3 Ⓐ Ⓑ Ⓒ Ⓓ Ⓔ	24 Ⓐ Ⓑ Ⓒ Ⓓ Ⓔ	45 Ⓐ Ⓑ Ⓒ Ⓓ Ⓔ	66 Ⓐ Ⓑ Ⓒ Ⓓ Ⓔ	87 Ⓐ Ⓑ Ⓒ Ⓓ Ⓔ
4 Ⓐ Ⓑ Ⓒ Ⓓ Ⓔ	25 Ⓐ Ⓑ Ⓒ Ⓓ Ⓔ	46 Ⓐ Ⓑ Ⓒ Ⓓ Ⓔ	67 Ⓐ Ⓑ Ⓒ Ⓓ Ⓔ	88 Ⓐ Ⓑ Ⓒ Ⓓ Ⓔ
5 Ⓐ Ⓑ Ⓒ Ⓓ Ⓔ	26 Ⓐ Ⓑ Ⓒ Ⓓ Ⓔ	47 Ⓐ Ⓑ Ⓒ Ⓓ Ⓔ	68 Ⓐ Ⓑ Ⓒ Ⓓ Ⓔ	89 Ⓐ Ⓑ Ⓒ Ⓓ Ⓔ
6 Ⓐ Ⓑ Ⓒ Ⓓ Ⓔ	27 Ⓐ Ⓑ Ⓒ Ⓓ Ⓔ	48 Ⓐ Ⓑ Ⓒ Ⓓ Ⓔ	69 Ⓐ Ⓑ Ⓒ Ⓓ Ⓔ	90 Ⓐ Ⓑ Ⓒ Ⓓ Ⓔ
7 Ⓐ Ⓑ Ⓒ Ⓓ Ⓔ	28 Ⓐ Ⓑ Ⓒ Ⓓ Ⓔ	49 Ⓐ Ⓑ Ⓒ Ⓓ Ⓔ	70 Ⓐ Ⓑ Ⓒ Ⓓ Ⓔ	91 Ⓐ Ⓑ Ⓒ Ⓓ Ⓔ
8 Ⓐ Ⓑ Ⓒ Ⓓ Ⓔ	29 Ⓐ Ⓑ Ⓒ Ⓓ Ⓔ	50 Ⓐ Ⓑ Ⓒ Ⓓ Ⓔ	71 Ⓐ Ⓑ Ⓒ Ⓓ Ⓔ	92 Ⓐ Ⓑ Ⓒ Ⓓ Ⓔ
9 Ⓐ Ⓑ Ⓒ Ⓓ Ⓔ	30 Ⓐ Ⓑ Ⓒ Ⓓ Ⓔ	51 Ⓐ Ⓑ Ⓒ Ⓓ Ⓔ	72 Ⓐ Ⓑ Ⓒ Ⓓ Ⓔ	93 Ⓐ Ⓑ Ⓒ Ⓓ Ⓔ
10 Ⓐ Ⓑ Ⓒ Ⓓ Ⓔ	31 Ⓐ Ⓑ Ⓒ Ⓓ Ⓔ	52 Ⓐ Ⓑ Ⓒ Ⓓ Ⓔ	73 Ⓐ Ⓑ Ⓒ Ⓓ Ⓔ	94 Ⓐ Ⓑ Ⓒ Ⓓ Ⓔ
11 Ⓐ Ⓑ Ⓒ Ⓓ Ⓔ	32 Ⓐ Ⓑ Ⓒ Ⓓ Ⓔ	53 Ⓐ Ⓑ Ⓒ Ⓓ Ⓔ	74 Ⓐ Ⓑ Ⓒ Ⓓ Ⓔ	95 Ⓐ Ⓑ Ⓒ Ⓓ Ⓔ
12 Ⓐ Ⓑ Ⓒ Ⓓ Ⓔ	33 Ⓐ Ⓑ Ⓒ Ⓓ Ⓔ	54 Ⓐ Ⓑ Ⓒ Ⓓ Ⓔ	75 Ⓐ Ⓑ Ⓒ Ⓓ Ⓔ	96 Ⓐ Ⓑ Ⓒ Ⓓ Ⓔ
13 Ⓐ Ⓑ Ⓒ Ⓓ Ⓔ	34 Ⓐ Ⓑ Ⓒ Ⓓ Ⓔ	55 Ⓐ Ⓑ Ⓒ Ⓓ Ⓔ	76 Ⓐ Ⓑ Ⓒ Ⓓ Ⓔ	97 Ⓐ Ⓑ Ⓒ Ⓓ Ⓔ
14 Ⓐ Ⓑ Ⓒ Ⓓ Ⓔ	35 Ⓐ Ⓑ Ⓒ Ⓓ Ⓔ	56 Ⓐ Ⓑ Ⓒ Ⓓ Ⓔ	77 Ⓐ Ⓑ Ⓒ Ⓓ Ⓔ	98 Ⓐ Ⓑ Ⓒ Ⓓ Ⓔ
15 Ⓐ Ⓑ Ⓒ Ⓓ Ⓔ	36 Ⓐ Ⓑ Ⓒ Ⓓ Ⓔ	57 Ⓐ Ⓑ Ⓒ Ⓓ Ⓔ	78 Ⓐ Ⓑ Ⓒ Ⓓ Ⓔ	99 Ⓐ Ⓑ Ⓒ Ⓓ Ⓔ
16 Ⓐ Ⓑ Ⓒ Ⓓ Ⓔ	37 Ⓐ Ⓑ Ⓒ Ⓓ Ⓔ	58 Ⓐ Ⓑ Ⓒ Ⓓ Ⓔ	79 Ⓐ Ⓑ Ⓒ Ⓓ Ⓔ	100 Ⓐ Ⓑ Ⓒ Ⓓ Ⓔ
17 Ⓐ Ⓑ Ⓒ Ⓓ Ⓔ	38 Ⓐ Ⓑ Ⓒ Ⓓ Ⓔ	59 Ⓐ Ⓑ Ⓒ Ⓓ Ⓔ	80 Ⓐ Ⓑ Ⓒ Ⓓ Ⓔ	101 Ⓐ Ⓑ Ⓒ Ⓓ Ⓔ
18 Ⓐ Ⓑ Ⓒ Ⓓ Ⓔ	39 Ⓐ Ⓑ Ⓒ Ⓓ Ⓔ	60 Ⓐ Ⓑ Ⓒ Ⓓ Ⓔ	81 Ⓐ Ⓑ Ⓒ Ⓓ Ⓔ	102 Ⓐ Ⓑ Ⓒ Ⓓ Ⓔ
19 Ⓐ Ⓑ Ⓒ Ⓓ Ⓔ	40 Ⓐ Ⓑ Ⓒ Ⓓ Ⓔ	61 Ⓐ Ⓑ Ⓒ Ⓓ Ⓔ	82 Ⓐ Ⓑ Ⓒ Ⓓ Ⓔ	103 Ⓐ Ⓑ Ⓒ Ⓓ Ⓔ
20 Ⓐ Ⓑ Ⓒ Ⓓ Ⓔ	41 Ⓐ Ⓑ Ⓒ Ⓓ Ⓔ	62 Ⓐ Ⓑ Ⓒ Ⓓ Ⓔ	83 Ⓐ Ⓑ Ⓒ Ⓓ Ⓔ	104 Ⓐ Ⓑ Ⓒ Ⓓ Ⓔ
21 Ⓐ Ⓑ Ⓒ Ⓓ Ⓔ	42 Ⓐ Ⓑ Ⓒ Ⓓ Ⓔ	63 Ⓐ Ⓑ Ⓒ Ⓓ Ⓔ	84 Ⓐ Ⓑ Ⓒ Ⓓ Ⓔ	105 Ⓐ Ⓑ Ⓒ Ⓓ Ⓔ